Diagnostic Handbook of
Otorhinolaryngology

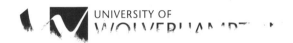

Diagnostic Handbook of
Otorhinolaryngology

Michael Hawke

MD, FRCS(C)
Professor of Otolaryngology, University of Toronto
Chief of Otolaryngology, St Joseph's Hospital, Toronto
Canada

Brian Bingham

MB ChB, FRCS
Honorary Senior Lecturer in Otolaryngology
University of Glasgow
Consultant ENT Surgeon, Victoria Infirmary, Glasgow
UK

Heinz Stammberger

MD
Professor of Otorhinolaryngology, University of Graz
Austria

Bruce Benjamin

OBE, DLO, FRACS, FAAP
Clinical Professor of Otorhinolaryngology
Sydney University
Australia

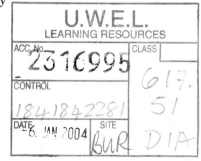
MARTIN DUNITZ

© 1997 Martin Dunitz Ltd, a member of the Taylor & Francis Group

First published in the United Kingdom in 1997

Paperback edition published in the United Kingdom in 2002 by
Martin Dunitz Ltd, The Livery House, 7–9 Pratt Street, London NW1 0AE

Tel.:   +44 (0) 20 74822202
Fax.:   +44 (0) 20 72670159
E-mail: info@dunitz.co.uk
Website: http://www.dunitz.co.uk

Portions of this book were originally published in 1995 as Bruce Benjamin,
Brian Bingham, Michael Hawke and Heinz Stammberger, *A Colour Atlas of
Otorhinolaryngology* (Martin Dunitz: London)

A CIP record for this book is available from the British Library.

ISBN 1 84184 228 1

Distributed in the USA by
Fulfilment Center
Taylor & Francis
7625 Empire Drive
Florence, KY 41042, USA
Toll Free Tel.: +1 800 634 7064
E-mail: cserve@routledge_ny.com

Distributed in Canada by
Taylor & Francis
74 Rolark Drive
Scarborough, Ontario M1R 4G2, Canada
Toll Free Tel.: +1 877 226 2237
E-mail: tal_fran@istar.ca

Distributed in the rest of the world by
Thomson Publishing Services
Cheriton House
North Way
Andover, Hampshire SP10 5BE, UK
Tel.: +44 (0)1264 332424
E-mail: salesorder.tandf@thomsonpublishingservices.co.uk

Composition by Scribe Design, Gillingham, Kent, UK
Printed and bound in Singapore by Kyodo Printing Co (S'pore) Pte Ltd

Contents

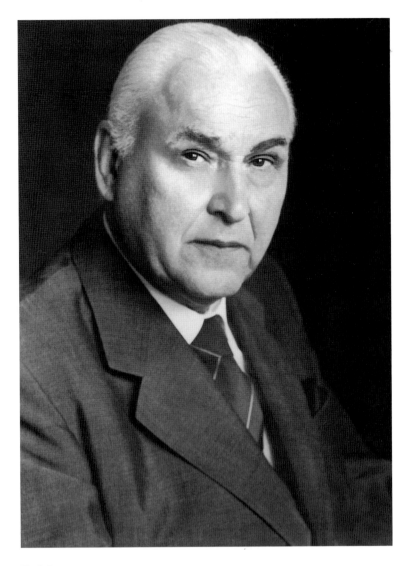

Karl Storz

1911–1996

This handbook is dedicated to the memory of Dr Karl Storz, without whose interest, encouragement and support, this and all other colour texts that require endoscopic colour photographs of the highest quality would not have been possible.

The authors would like to take this opportunity to pay tribute to the memory of Dr Karl Storz. Born in 1911, he served a three-year apprenticeship at his father's company, becoming an instrument maker. During this time he learned to appreciate the need for high-quality surgical instruments. At the conclusion of his apprenticeship Karl Storz became aware that he needed more experience in order to be able to cover the entire range of medical equipment, and for this reason he followed up his initial training by working for several years at a well known medical-supply company in Leipzig. His experience during this time formed the basis for his later work: in particular, his exposure to instruments from many different manufacturers, which he meticulously analysed, and his direct contact with numerous physicians and surgeons expanded both his knowledge of the art of instrument making and also his understanding of the problems that physicians had with the existing instruments. His realization that these problems could only be solved by close contact between the physician and the instrument manufacturer—which was not a common practice in those days—became one of the most important factors in his success: this close relationship with the medical practitioner bore fruit right from the onset and soon led to developments that were to have a lasting effect on the world of endoscopy.

In 1945, with his father's assistance, Karl Storz founded the present firm of Karl Storz GmbH in Tuttlingen, southern Germany. Initially, the firm made specialized instruments in collaboration with several important European physicians, including Kleinsasser, Messerklinger, and Maasen. The firm subsequently expanded into the field of bronchoscopy, which at that time was primarily concerned with the removal of inhaled foreign bodies.

By the end of the 1940s Karl Storz had designed his own optical system and produced optical and flexible forceps for use with the rigid bronchoscopes. In 1956 he successfully developed an extracorporeal flash unit. Later he realized that light could be transmitted with the aid of glass fibres. This was the dawn of 'cold light' endoscopy. Subsequently a new light source was developed which contained an integral flash tube for photo documentation.

In 1966 Karl Storz recognized the value of the Hopkins rod lens system which was designed by Professor Harold Hopkins of the University of Reading in the United Kingdom. The introduction of these new Hopkins rod lens telescopes revolutionized the entire field of endoscopy and set a new 'benchmark' for endoscopic image transmission. The combination of 'cold light' illumination, Hopkins rod endoscopes and the introduction of outstanding photodocumentation equipment led to a sustained period of rapid growth in Karl Storz GmbH. Production now embraced every specialized medical field for adults, children, and infants; in addition, Karl Storz endoscopes and fibreoptic telescopes were used in engine construction, air and space travel, architecture and archaeology.

There were three key factors that contributed to the success of his young company: his precise knowledge of the requirements of the end user, which was based upon dialogue with the physician; combined with a craftsman's ability to solve problems as simply but as effectively as possible; and his understanding and support of those individuals who by their ideas were capable of providing a vital contribution to the further development of optical and technical systems. The outstanding contributions of Karl Storz to the field of medicine and medical instrument manufacture were recognized by the University of Marburg, which awarded him a Doctorate of Medicine.

In the field of Ear, Nose and Throat–Head and Neck Surgery, photographic documentation is of supreme importance: it provides an objective, natural-coloured record with accurate detail which is eminently suitable for teaching. The Karl Storz Hopkins telescopes, with their rigid glass rod lens system, provide the examiner with a magnified, clear, full-coloured, wide angled image with unlimited photographic capabilities. The authors of this handbook all use Karl Storz photographic equipment, and the majority of the photographs in this handbook were taken with Karl Storz state-of-the-art photographic equipment.

In 1996, with the death of Dr Karl Storz, the medical community lost one of its pre-eminent instrument manufacturers, supporters and friends.

Preface

Pluris est oculatus testis unus quam auriti decem;
qui audiunt audita dicunt, qui vident plane sciunt.

('One eye-witness is worth more than ten relying on hearsay;
those who hear can only repeat what they have heard, but those
who see have real knowledge')

Plautus, *Truculentus* II. vi
(second century BC)

The establishment of any 'diagnosis' is a complex professional
exercise that is a mandatory prelude to the rational management
of the disease process. While the clinical features of a patient's
history may suggest a possible diagnosis, definitive identification
(diagnosis) of diseases is often dependent upon specific signs
elicited by visual inspection; nowhere is this more important
than in the field of otorhinolaryngology.

Examination of the ear, the nasal cavity, the nasopharynx, the
oropharynx, the larynx, the tracheo-bronchial tree and the
oesophagus has in the past depended primarily on naked eye
examination. Today, with modern technology, the search for
visual diagnostic clues now relies most commonly on sophisti-
cated optical systems, including the fibreoptic halogen otoscope,
the flexible fibreoptic nasopharyngolaryngoscope, the rigid rod
lens telescope and in some cases the operating microscope.

This handbook has been prepared primarily for those general
practitioners, nurse practitioners and medical students who
diagnose and treat diseases of the ear, nose, throat and neck.
We hope that those who use this handbook will find it a valuable
addition to their library and to their 'visual database'.

Michael Hawke
Brian Bingham
Heinz Stammberger
Bruce Benjamin

Acknowledgements

The authors are grateful to the following for permission to reproduce figures:

Dr CT Buiter (Figure 2.84);
Dr B Fisher (Figure 1.42);
Dr MA Knowling and the Editor of the *Canadian Medical Association Journal* (Figure 1.17);
Dr S Krajden (Figure 1.34);
Dr M May (Figure 2.16, top);
Dr DP Mitchell (Figure 1.51);
Dr L Shankar (Figure 1.116).

1 The ear

Introduction

The ear is divided into four anatomical areas: the external ear, the external auditory canal, the middle ear and the inner ear. This chapter concentrates on disorders of the outer three parts of the ear, where a diagnosis can often be made on inspection.

The pinna

The external ear (also called the 'auricle' or 'pinna') is composed of fibroelastic cartilage covered by skin. In humans it has only a minor role to play in sound localization and sound amplification; it also protects the external ear canal. The pinna, as the result of its exposed position, is liable to damage by the wind, cold, sunlight and local trauma. Skin disorders frequently affect the pinna, and a sound knowledge of dermatology is therefore helpful. In any examination of the pinna all areas must be inspected, and the examiner must never forget to 'look behind the ear'.

The external auditory canal

The external auditory canal commences at the medial end of the conchal bowl and extends medially to the tympanic membrane to provide a passage through which the airborne sound waves collected at the pinna are transmitted to the tympanic membrane. Anatomically and pathologically the lateral surface of the tympanic membrane is considered part of the external auditory canal. The tympanic membrane is set at an oblique angle to the ear canal, with the anterior canal wall measuring approximately 30 mm in length and the posterior canal wall measuring approximately 25 mm in length. A great deal of protection is provided for the tympanic membrane by the length and convoluted shape of the external auditory canal.

The external auditory canal has an efficient self–cleaning mechanism that results from the continuous migration of epithelium from the deep meatus to the outer part of the canal where the keratin squames are shed. Many disorders affecting the external auditory canal result from either failure of or trauma to the normal self-cleansing mechanism of the canal epithelium. Trauma to the epithelium arises commonly from the insertion of foreign objects into the canal, and the advice to any patient should be that 'if you want to put something in your ear — try your elbow!'

The middle ear

The middle ear transmits sound waves from the tympanic membrane to the inner ear. The middle ear cleft (the tubotympanic cavity) commences at the nasopharyngeal opening of the eustachian tube. There are three major components to the middle ear cleft: the middle ear cavity proper (which contains the three ossicles), the eustachian tube (which provides a source of ventilation and pressure equalization) and the mastoid air cell system (whose precise function is unknown). Proper functioning of the eustachian tube is essential for the maintenance of aeration and the normal functioning of the middle ear; indeed, malfunction of the eustachian tube is the principal cause of most disorders of the middle ear.

The anterior half of the middle ear is lined by a respiratory ciliated type of epithelium which contains two types of mucus-producing cells. The mucus produced by these glands provides protection and lubrication for the respiratory mucoperiosteum which is exposed to the air within the middle ear. Mucociliary flow is the major defence mechanism of this respiratory epithelium and the role of the mucous blanket in this system is crucial. In the absence of sufficient or normal mucus, the mucociliary clearance system fails.

Pinna

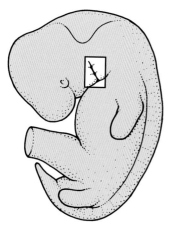 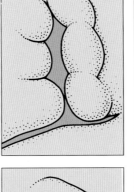 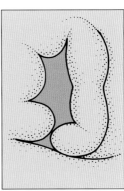

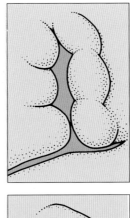 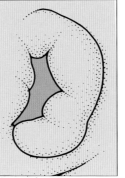 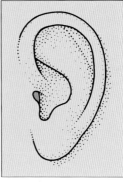

Figure 1.1
Embryology of auricle

The pinna or external auricle is formed from six hillocks that arise on either side of the dorsal extremity of the first branchial groove between 4 and 6 weeks of gestation. These hillocks are gradually transformed into the complex folds of the fully formed auricle.

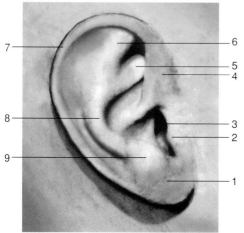

Figure 1.2
Surface anatomy of pinna

The common surface landmarks of the pinna are as follows: 1, lobule; 2, tragus; 3, external auditory canal; 4, crus of the helix; 5, inferior crus of the antihelix; 6, superior crus; 7, helix; 8, antihelix; 9, antitragus. While the relative proportion of the structures varies from individual to individual, their presence is relatively constant.

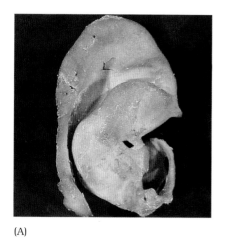

(A)

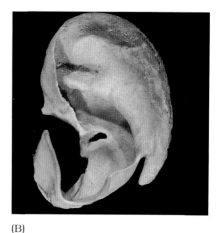

(B)

Figure 1.3
Cartilaginous framework of pinna

The shape of the external ear is determined by the configuration of the underlying cartilaginous skeleton. This illustration shows a cadaveric cartilage dissection from both (A) the medial and (B) the lateral aspects.

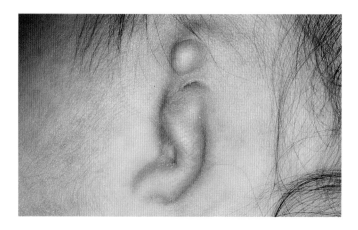

Figure 1.4
Microtia

The term 'microtia' is used when there is gross underdevelopment of the pinna with a blind or absent external auditory canal. It is important to remember that congenital malformations of the external ear are frequently associated with malformations of other portions of the ear or face.

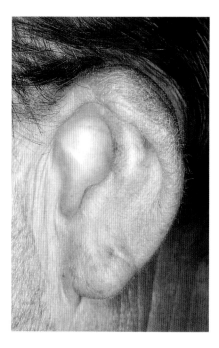

Figure 1.5
Atresia

In this patient there is a partial atresia of the pinna and a complete atresia of the external auditory canal.

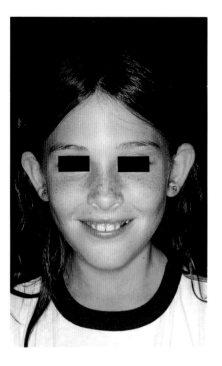

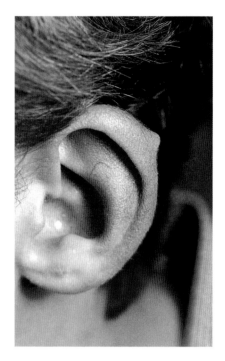

Figure 1.6
Outstanding ear

Minor deformities of the helix and
antihelix are the most common
malformations of the external ear.
When the angle between the auricle
and the side of the head is greater
than normal, the result is an
outstanding ear. Outstanding ears
are inherited by means of an
autosomal dominant gene with
complete penetrance and variable
expressivity.

Figure 1.7
Darwin's tubercle

A Darwin's tubercle is a small
cartilaginous protuberance most
commonly situated along the concave
edge of the posterosuperior helix and
usually projecting anteriorly.
Occasionally, and more obviously, a
Darwin's tubercle will project
posteriorly, as shown in this
illustration. Cosmetic removal of such
a tubercle may be required to avoid
the childhood taunt of 'pixie ear'. A
Darwin's tubercle is inherited by
means of an autosomal dominant
gene with variable expressivity.

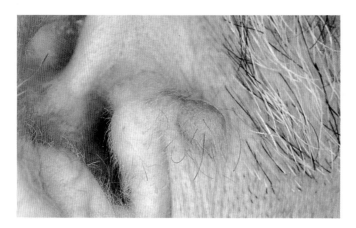

Figure 1.8
Preauricular tag

Preauricular tags are small congenital pedunculated projections arising from the skin of the face just in front of the pinna; the most common location for a preauricular tag is just anterior to the upper border of the tragus.

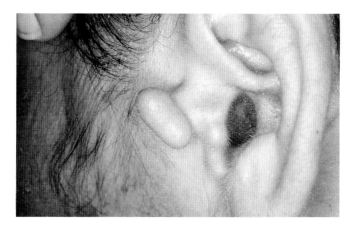

Figure 1.9
Accessory auricle

A preauricular appendage that contains a cartilaginous core is called an 'accessory auricle'. Accessory auricles represent a small ectopic remnant of one of the six embryological hillocks from which the pinna is formed.

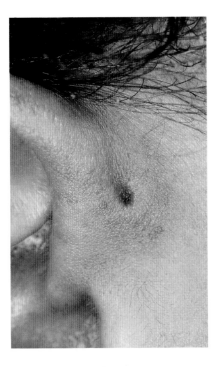

Figure 1.10
Preauricular pit

Preauricular pits are shallow pits that result either from a failure in the fusion of the primitive ear hillocks or from the defective closure of the first branchial cleft. They are most characteristically located in, or just in front of, the anterior crus of the helix. Preauricular pits are inherited through an autosomal dominant gene with incomplete penetrance.

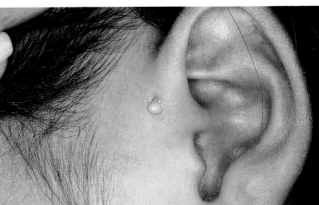

Figure 1.11
Infected preauricular sinus

A preauricular sinus is deeper than a preauricular pit. The sinus tract is lined with a stratified squamous or columnar epithelium and may become chronically infected, emitting a painless, foul-smelling, milky discharge.

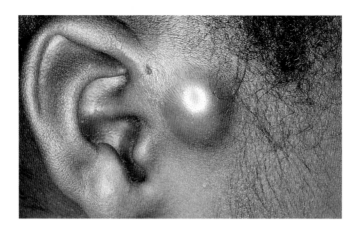

Figure 1.12
Preauricular cyst

If the external opening of the tract of a preauricular sinus becomes obstructed, the epithelium lining the tract will continue to shed epithelial squames into the tract, thereby producing a preauricular cyst.

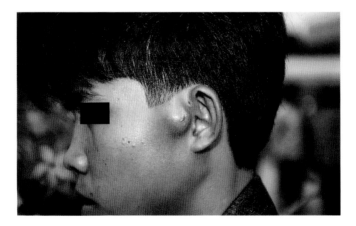

Figure 1.13
Infected preauricular cyst

When an infection develops in a preauricular sinus, it is usually more acute and associated with pain and swelling. Since there is no external connection in a preauricular sinus, a mini-abscess usually forms, which, if left untreated, will eventually drain from the sinus through the skin.

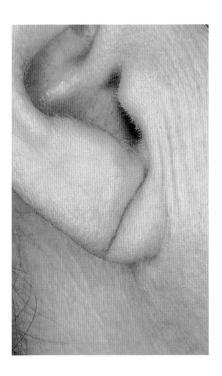

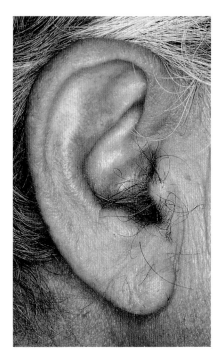

Figure 1.14
Creased lobule

In some individuals an oblique crease may appear in the skin of the lobule with increasing age. This is known as a 'creased lobule' and is associated with a predisposition to obstructive coronary artery disease.

Figure 1.15
Hairy tragus

With age, coarse hairs may appear on the male tragus. This secondary sex characteristic is known as a 'hairy tragus'. It is interesting to note that the word 'tragus' is derived from the Greek *tragos* (goat), which alludes to the resemblance of these hairs to a goat's beard.

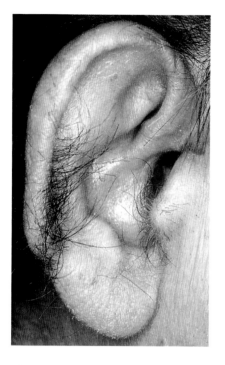

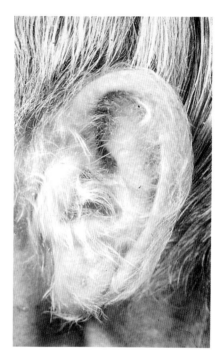

Figure 1.16
Hairy pinna

The development of coarse hairs over
the pinna is known as a 'hairy
pinna'. These coarse hairs most
commonly appear over the lower
portion of the helix. Hairy pinna
occurs only in males and is a Y-
linked trait whose expression
increases with age.

Figure 1.17
Hypertrichosis lanuginosa acquisita

'Hypertrichosis lanuginosa acquisita'
is the term applied to the excessive
growth of fine hair of the lanugus or
vellus type. Hypertrichosis lanuginosa
acquisita is associated with the use
of certain medicines such as
phenytoin, streptomycin,
penicillamine and minoxidil. Certain
metabolic conditions, including
porphyria, pregnancy,
hyperthyroidism, and malnutrition,
and occasionally the presence of
malignant disease have also been
associated with this condition.
(Reproduced with the kind
permission of Dr MA Knowling and
the Editor of the *Canadian Medical
Association Journal*.)

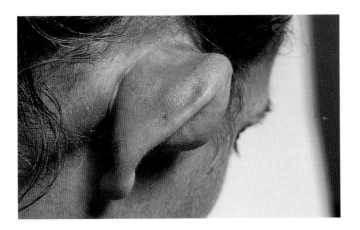

Figure 1.18
Haematoma

A haematoma of the pinna is usually the result of blunt trauma
sustained during such activities as boxing or wrestling. If the trauma
tears one of the small vessels that lie between the perichondrium and
the underlying auricular cartilage, then blood will collect in the
subperichondrial plane, thereby elevating the perichondrium from the
underlying cartilage. The loose subcutaneous tissue between the skin
and the perichondrium on the medial aspect of the auricle usually
provides considerable mobility, and as a result a haematoma will form
less commonly on the medial surface of the auricle unless the
auricular cartilage has been fractured.

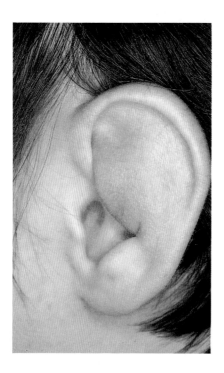

Figure 1.19
Traumatic seroma

Chronic trauma from friction may irritate the perichondrium and produce a subperichondrial serous or serosanguineous collection of fluid called a 'seroma'. A seroma will usually persist for several days after the original injury.

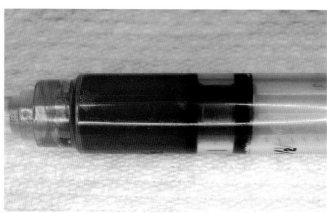

Figure 1.20
Traumatic seroma

Should a seroma fail to resolve spontaneously, aspiration of the subperichondrial blood-tinged serous transudate may be necessary.

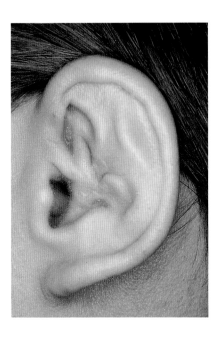

**Figure 1.21
Cauliflower ear**

Severe or repeated trauma to the auricle may produce areas of subperichondrial separation, shearing and localized haemorrhage, which result in devitalization of the underlying cartilage. This devitalization and its associated healing process may produce excessive subcutaneous fibrous tissue and scar formation, which deform the surface of the pinna.

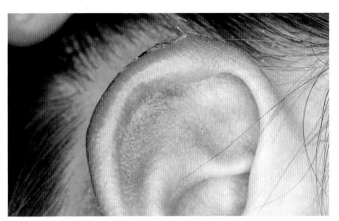

**Figure 1.22
Solar dermatitis**

The superior portion of the pinna is susceptible to acute solar damage (sunburn). The superior portion of this pinna shows erythema, oedema and blistering, which are the result of a 'second-degree' sunburn. As will be seen later, repeated solar damage predisposes an individual to premalignant and malignant cutaneous changes.

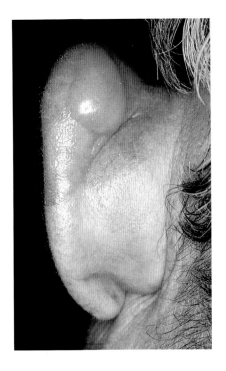

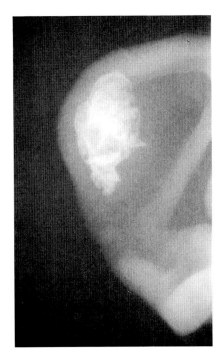

Figure 1.23
Frostbite

Tissue damage from extreme cold is
similar in appearance to that
sustained from heat injuries. Note
the large serous-filled bulla with
oedema of the surrounding skin. This
is a 'second-degree' frostbite.

Figure 1.24
**Frostbite-induced calcification of
auricular cartilage**

The soft-tissue radiograph of the
pinna of this patient who had severe
frostbite many years previously
revealed extensive calcification
throughout the posterior superior
portion of the auricular cartilage.
This was clinically manifest as a
hard 'bony' pinna.

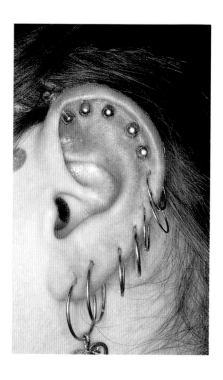

Figure 1.25
Multiple earrings

'Beauty is in the eye of the beholder'. Some individuals favour wearing more than one earring in each ear. The upper five earrings in this patient have penetrated through the auricular cartilage and thus predispose the patient to perichondritis.

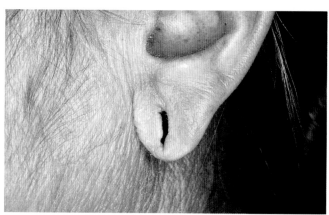

Figure 1.26
Elongated earring hole

Years of traction from a heavy earring have gradually elongated the hole in this lobule.

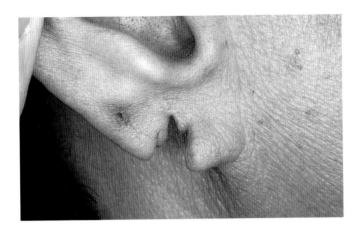

Figure 1.27
Traumatic split lobule

The irregular cut-out deformity in this lobule was the result of the traumatic avulsion of an earring. Such injuries usually occur when a large hoop type of earring is accidentally grasped and pulled by an infant or young child.

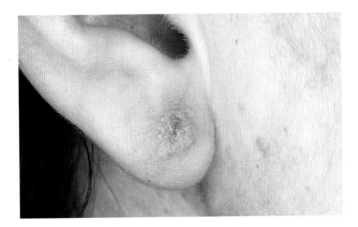

Figure 1.28
Infected earring tract

Localized infections within the earring tract are usually the result of poor hygiene. In these patients pressure on the lobule will frequently expel a tiny drop of pus.

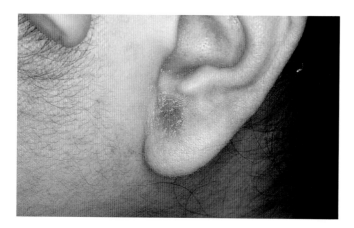

Figure 1.29
Contact dermatitis

The red and excoriated area around the earring tract in the lobule of
this patient was the result of a nickel contact dermatitis.

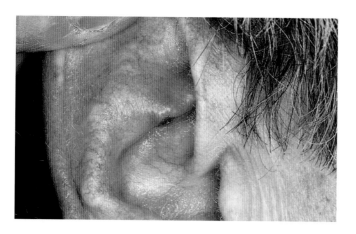

Figure 1.30
Ear mould pressure atrophy

Long-standing pressure from a poorly fitting ear mould has caused
ulceration of the upper portion of the antitragus.

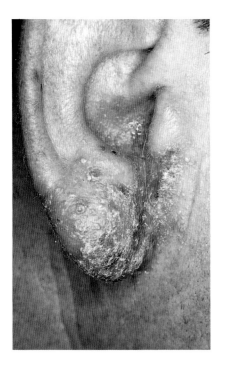

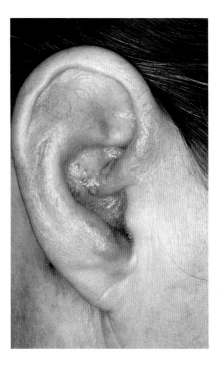

Figure 1.31
Contact dermatitis

Contact dermatitis of the external ear is relatively common and may be confused with infectious otitis externa; patients with contact dermatitis complain primarily of itching rather than pain. A neomycin-containing ointment has produced in this patient an erythematous, weeping allergic reaction which has extended on to the skin of the neck where the offending medication has tracked.

Figure 1.32
Herpes zoster (shingles)

Herpes zoster is an acute localized viral infection of the skin caused by the varicella-zoster virus. This large DNA-containing virus of the herpes-virus group causes, in the early stage, scattered pustules in the skin of the involved sensory dermatome.

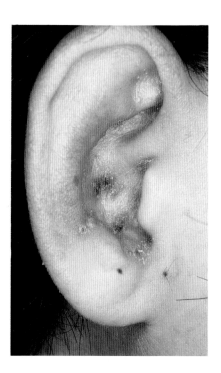

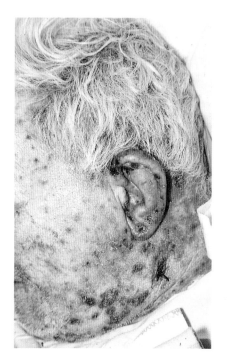

Figure 1.33
Herpes zoster (shingles)

Over time the pustules rupture, dry out and become crusted. When herpes zoster involves the sensory portion of the geniculate ganglion of the facial nerve, it may produce a lower motor neuron facial paralysis and associated herpetic eruption over the affected dermatomes. This is called the Ramsay Hunt syndrome (herpes zoster oticus).

Figure 1.34
Disseminated herpes zoster

In patients with a deficient immune defence system, such as this patient with leukaemia, herpes zoster infection may spread dramatically. (Courtesy of Dr S Krajden.)

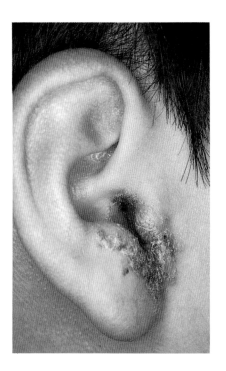

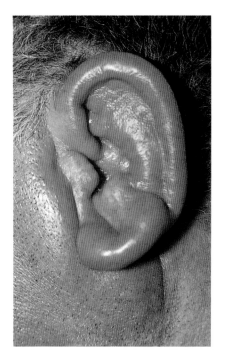

Figure 1.35
Impetigo contagiosa

The *Staphylococcus aureus*-laden
discharge from the middle ear of this
patient has caused a localized
superficial infective dermatitis
(impetigo) over the upper portion of
the lobule. Ulcerative impetigo is a
result of a deeper bacterial skin
infection—most commonly group A
streptococci, staphylococci or a
mixture of these bacteria. Note the
ulceration in the postauricular crease
of this patient.

Figure 1.36
Erysipelas

Erysipelas is an acute, localized but
spreading superficial cellulitis usually
caused by group A beta haemolytic
streptococci and characterized by
involvement of the lymphatics. The
cutaneous lesions are bright red, well
demarcated and tender, with an
elevated and distinct advancing
peripheral margin.

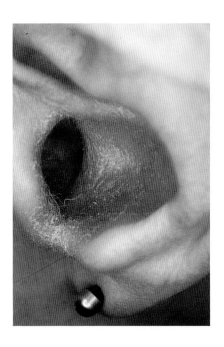

Figure 1.37
Chronic dermatitis

While healthy skin normally provides an effective physical and chemical barrier against the numerous bacteria and fungi to which it is constantly exposed, under conditions of trauma, moisture or maceration this effective antimicrobial barrier may break down. The result may be a chronic infective dermatitis caused by bacteria, fungi or a mixture of both. The diffuse dermatitis throughout this patient's conchal bowl is the result of infection by *Staphylococcus aureus* and *Candida albicans* secondary to the wearing of a hearing aid ear mould.

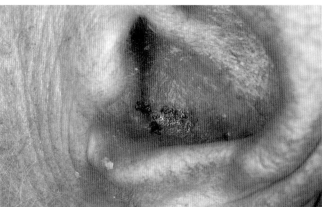

Figure 1.38
Neurodermatitis

Itching is a common feature in patients with chronic dermatitis and repeated scratching of the pruritic area may break down the skin barrier, allowing dermatitis to develop further. The term 'neurodermatitis' has been applied to these patients in whom telltale areas of excoriation or bleeding are frequently seen. This vicious cycle of itching, scratching, infection and more itching may be very difficult to break.

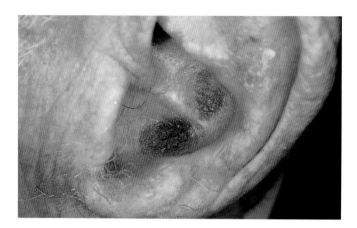

Figure 1.39
Neglect keratosis

Sheets of keratin squames are constantly pushed up to the surface of the skin and shed during normal epidermal maintenance. The outermost layer of squames (the stratum corneum) is normally rubbed away by contact with clothing or as a result of personal toilet. Neglected areas of skin may accumulate patches of thick keratin debris, resulting in a pigmented, greasy, raised lesion that at first glance resembles an area of seborrhoeic keratosis. Unlike seborrhoeic keratosis, these areas of neglect keratosis are easily removed with a cotton-tipped applicator to reveal normal underlying skin.

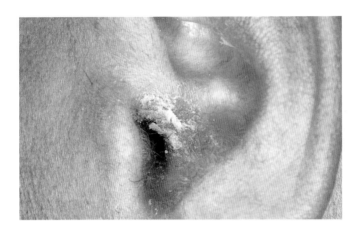

Figure 1.40
Psoriasis vulgaris

Psoriasis vulgaris is a hereditary disorder of skin characterized by an increased rate of epidermal cell replication. Note the sharply demarcated, salmon-coloured plaques of psoriasis just below the helical rim. The upper portion of the lesion is covered with the characteristic silvery scales.

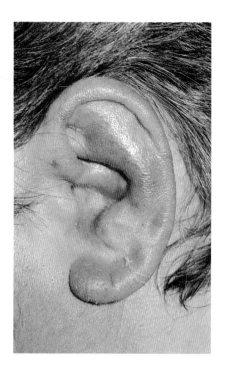

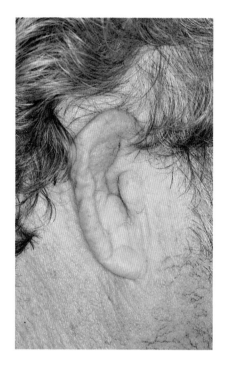

Figure 1.41
Acute perichondritis

Acute perichondritis is caused by a bacterial infection of the perichondrium, which is usually the result of trauma to the pinna. Acute perichondritis most commonly occurs following lacerations or incisions that extend through the perichondrium. Clinically, the skin of the pinna is diffusely swollen, painful and tender.

Figure 1.42
Relapsing polychondritis

Relapsing polychondritis is an episodic and generally progressive inflammation of the cartilaginous structures of the body. An autoimmune aetiology is suspected since many of these patients have circulating antibodies to type II collagen (the collagen present in cartilage). Clinically, relapsing polychondritis is characterized by bilateral auricular chondritis, nasal chondritis, laryngeal chondritis, polyarthritis and respiratory tract chondritis. Ocular inflammation may also be present. (Courtesy of Dr B Fisher.)

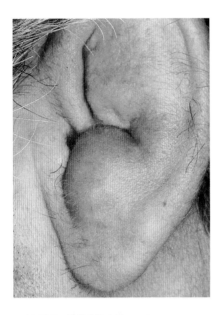

Figure 1.43
Idiopathic cystic chondromalacia of external auricular cartilage

Benign idiopathic cystic chondromalacia (auricular pseudocyst) is a cystic degeneration of the auricular cartilage of unknown origin, which may be mistaken both clinically and histologically for relapsing polychondritis. Clinically, this disease presents as an isolated, unilateral, asymptomatic swelling, most commonly on the anterior surface of the pinna. These pseudocysts may be the result of repeated local minor trauma to the auricular cartilage. Aspiration of a pseudocyst will produce a yellow or orange serous fluid.

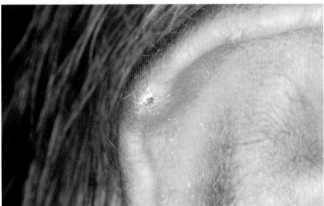

Figure 1.44
Chondrodermatitis nodularis helicis chronica (Winkler's nodule)

Chondrodermatitis nodularis helicis chronica is the formal name given to a discrete, firm, raised and frequently painful nodule, most commonly located on the apex of the helix of the ear. This disease appears to be the result of solar damage to the underlying cartilage, which undergoes degeneration and extrusion through the skin. These lesions are exquisitely tender to the touch. Local excision of the overlying skin and underlying auricular cartilage is curative.

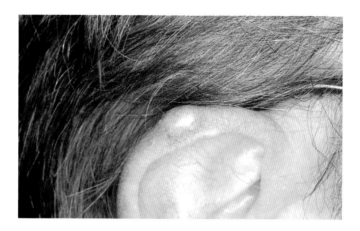

Figure 1.45
Gouty tophi

Gouty tophi are the result of the subcutaneous accumulation of deposits of monosodium urate crystals. These tophi present as painful, skin-covered nodules occurring most frequently on the helix. Tophi are gritty to palpation and the underlying yellow crystals may occasionally be seen through the skin.

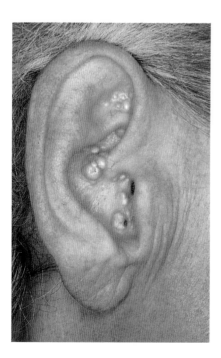

Figure 1.46
Milia

Milia are multiple, superficially located, small white cysts that arise from the lowest portion of the infundibulum in the region of the sebaceous duct. These tiny cysts differ from epidermal cysts only in size.

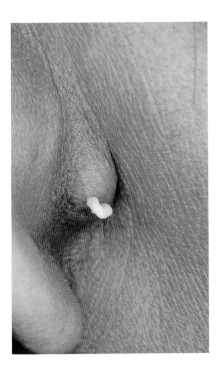

Figure 1.47
Epidermal cyst

Epidermal cysts are slow-growing, round, firm intradermal or subcutaneous cysts that arise most commonly from the infundibulum of a hair follicle.

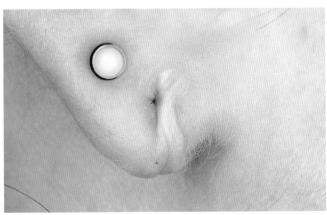

Figure 1.48
Hypertrophic scar

Hypertrophic scars are raised scars that remain within the confines of the wound and usually flatten spontaneously over 1–2 years.

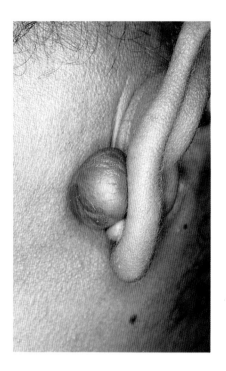 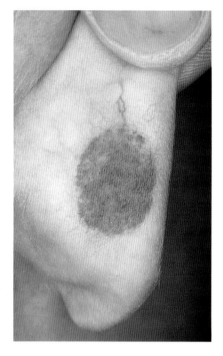

Figure 1.49
Keloid

Keloids are abnormal scars which not only persist but also extend beyond the site of the original injury. Keloids occur more often in Blacks than in Whites and are most frequent in the second and third decades of life.

Figure 1.50
Capillary haemangioma

Capillary haemangioma or strawberry birthmark is a bright red, soft, lobulated, benign tumour consisting of numerous blood-filled, benign-looking capillaries. Seventy per cent of capillary haemangiomas undergo spontaneous resolution in the first decade of life.

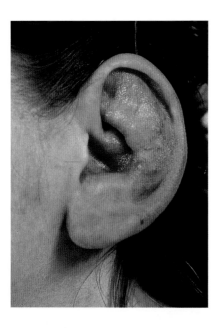

Figure 1.51
Arteriovenous malformation

Arteriovenous malformations may involve the blood vessels within the pinna. Clinically, an arteriovenous malformation will present with discolouration and distortion of the skin overlying the pinna. Palpation of the involved area will reveal pulsations, and auscultation will reveal a loud bruit. (Courtesy of Dr DP Mitchell.)

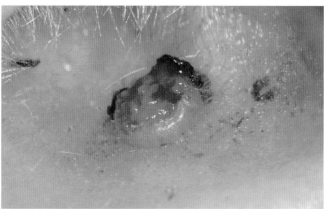

Figure 1.52
Keratoacanthoma

A keratoacanthoma is a benign, usually solitary, rapidly developing epithelial neoplasm that arises on the sun-exposed areas of fair-skinned, elderly individuals. The lesion is characterized by a firm, dome-shaped nodule with skin-coloured rolled edges and a central crater filled with keratin debris, which clinically and histologically resembles a squamous cell carcinoma. Because of its resemblance to squamous cell carcinoma, a biopsy is indicated.

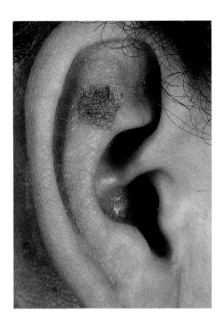

Figure 1.53
Seborrhoeic keratosis

Seborrhoeic keratoses are benign tumours that appear after the third decade of life. Clinically, they appear as raised, greasy, 'stuck-on' lesions with visible keratotic plugs filling a central irregular crypt. Seborrhoeic keratosis may vary in colour from light yellow through brown to black with the intensity of the colour varying with the amount of melanin pigment present in the lesion. When examined with a magnifying glass, keratin or horn cysts can be seen on the surface of the lesion.

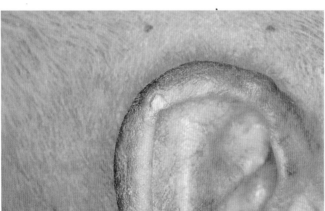

Figure 1.54
Solar keratosis (actinic keratosis or senile keratosis)

Solar keratoses are premalignant lesions that arise on sun-exposed areas of the skin. Clinically, solar keratoses appear as dry, rough and adherent scaly lesions. Occasionally, solar keratoses produce a circumscribed, conical, hyperkeratotic excrescence, which is known as a cutaneous horn. A solar keratosis is considered to be premalignant as it may develop into a squamous cell carcinoma.

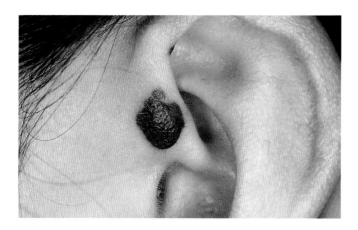

Figure 1.55
Intradermal naevus

This raised, pigmented, dome-shaped lesion on the upper border of the tragus is an intradermal naevus.

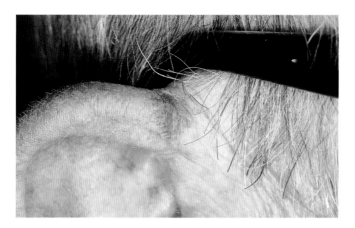

Figure 1.56
Solar lentigo

Solar lentigo is another lesion that develops from repeated exposure to the sun. These lesions rarely occur before the fourth decade of life, slowly increasing in both size and number. Clinically, solar lentigo appears as multiple, uniformly pigmented, dark-brown, flat lesions with an irregular outline.

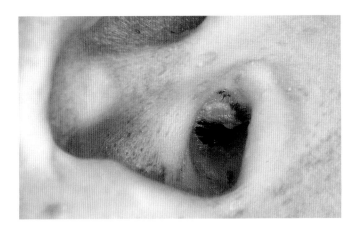

Figure 1.57
Verruca vulgaris

Verruca vulgaris or the common wart is a benign, localized area of epithelial hyperplasia caused by the human wart virus of the papova-virus group. Verrucae appear as firm, circumscribed elevated papules with a filiform or papillomatous and hyperkeratotic surface.

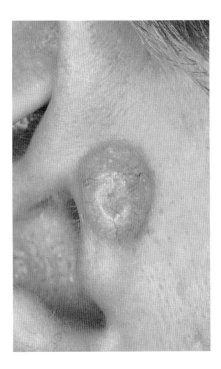

Figure 1.58
Basal cell carcinoma

Basal cell carcinoma is the most common cutaneous malignancy. These tumours usually develop in skin that has been subject to actinic damage, and it is therefore not surprising that basal cell carcinomas are the most common malignant tumour affecting the external ear. Basal cell carcinomas may present with many different clinical appearances. Any chronically ulcerated or raised lesion that persists should be biopsied.

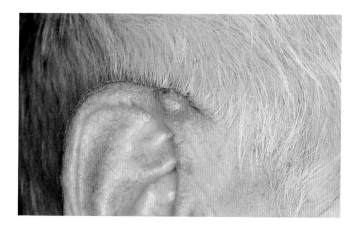

Figure 1.59
Squamous cell carcinoma

Squamous cell carcinoma of the auricle is a relatively uncommon
malignant tumour that arises from keratinocytes damaged by exposure to
sunlight. The diagnosis of a squamous cell carcinoma is made by biopsy.
As with basal cell carcinoma, any lesion that does not heal or shows any
suggestion of invasion of the underlying tissues should be biopsied.

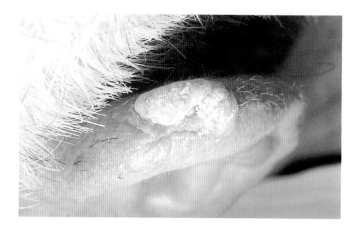

Figure 1.60
Verrucous carcinoma

Verrucous carcinoma is a low-grade squamous cell carcinoma that is slow
growing and initially exophytic and wart-like in appearance. Verrucous
carcinoma is characterized by slow and continual advancement with a
special predisposition for destruction of adjacent bony structures.

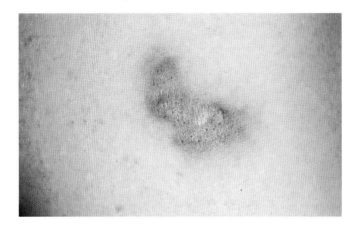

Figure 1.61
Kaposi's sarcoma

Kaposi's sarcoma is a sarcoma of vascular cell origin whose incidence
has increased dramatically as a result of the worldwide epidemic of
acquired immune deficiency syndrome (AIDS). Kaposi's sarcoma
usually presents as a raised purplish-red nodule that continues to
expand and enlarge. The diagnosis is made by biopsy. Diagnosis of
Kaposi's sarcoma strongly raises the possibility of HIV-positive
status.

External auditory canal

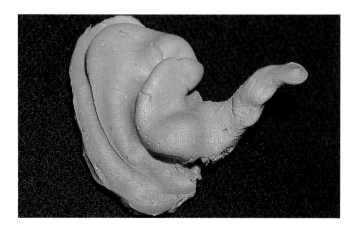

Figure 1.62
Normal superficial external auditory canal

The external auditory canal connecting the tympanic membrane to the exterior via the conchal bowl is divided into three distinct sections: the external or cartilaginous section, the medial or bony section and the lateral surface of the tympanic membrane. The shape of the external auditory canal and its relationship to the conchal bowl of the pinna are shown in this postmortem impression.

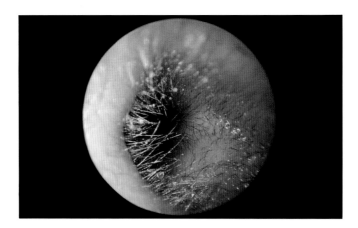

Figure 1.63
Cartilaginous portion of the external auditory canal

The skin lining the outer or cartilaginous portion of the external auditory canal is thick, hair-bearing skin containing numerous sebaceous and ceruminous glands. The cartilaginous portion of the external canal is relatively strong and mobile and is supported within a surrounding cartilaginous framework. (Right ear)

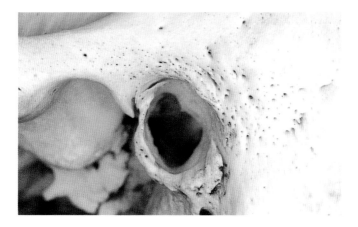

Figure 1.64
Bony external auditory canal

The medial (deep) or bony portion of the external auditory canal is surrounded by a bony framework, which consists primarily of the U-shaped tympanic bone. (Left ear)

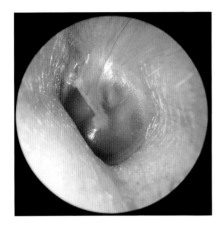

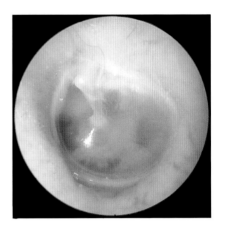

Figure 1.65
Bony external auditory canal

The skin lining the bony portion of
the external auditory canal is thin
and lacks adnexal structures, i.e.
hairs and glands. It is firmly
attached to the surrounding bony
framework. (Left ear)

Figure 1.66
Tympanic membrane

The external auditory canal ends at
the tympanic membrane. The
tympanic membrane appears as a
pale-grey, semi-transparent
membrane positioned obliquely at the
medial end of the external auditory
canal. (Left ear)

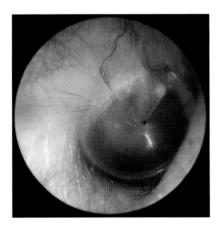

Figure 1.67
Epithelial migration 1

The normal self-cleansing of the
external auditory canal is the result
of the miraculous ability of the
epithelium lining the canal to migrate
in an outward direction. In this
volunteer an ink dot has been
applied to the surface of the
tympanic membrane in the region of
the umbo in order to demonstrate
this phenomenon. (Right ear)

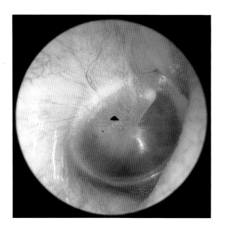

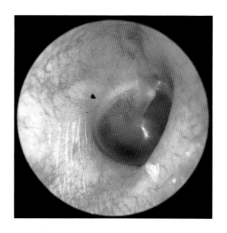

Figure 1.68
Epithelial migration 2

Two months later the ink dot has migrated in a radial or centrifugal direction over the surface of the tympanic membrane to a position overlying the area of the incudostapedial joint. (Right ear)

Figure 1.69
Epithelial migration 3

A further 2 months later the ink dot has migrated on to the bony external auditory canal in the 10 o'clock position. (Right ear)

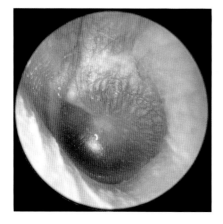

Figure 1.70
Keratin patches on tympanic membrane

Small, radially orientated patches of thickened keratin squames can often be seen on the surface of the normal tympanic membrane. These patches consist of older and thicker keratin from the central portion of the tympanic membrane which have migrated centrifugally. (Left ear)

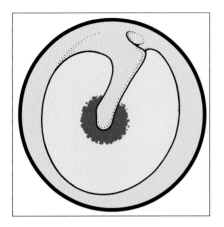

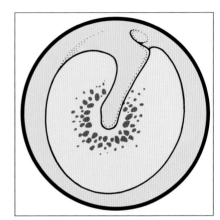

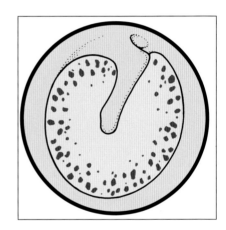

Figure 1.71
Keratin patches on tympanic membrane

As the superficial keratin layer of the central portion of the tympanic membrane migrates centrifugally, it must also spread laterally to cover the widened peripheral areas of the drum, resulting in the development of separation lines.

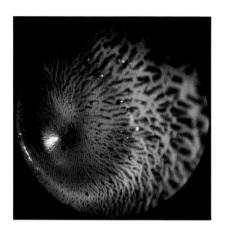

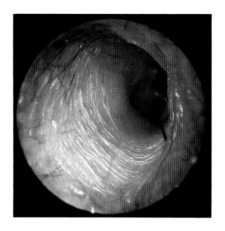

Figure 1.72
Keratin patches on tympanic membrane: osmium staining

The shape, size and number of keratin patches can be clearly seen in this cadaveric specimen in which the keratin patches have been emphasized by staining with osmium tetroxide. (Left ear)

Figure 1.73
Transverse epithelial wrinkles

Transverse wrinkles are superficial waves or corrugations that lie at right angles to the long axis of the external auditory canal. These wrinkles are present in most external canals and are most readily visible in the epithelium covering the posterior bony canal wall. These transverse wrinkles develop as the outwardly migrating stratum corneum of the deep canal becomes heaped up against the pressure of the stationary hairs of the superficial canal. (Right ear)

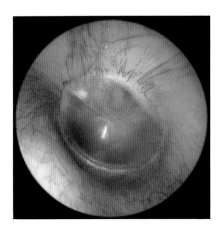

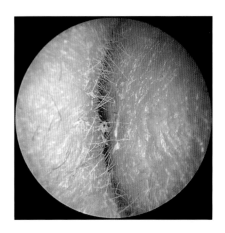

Figure 1.74
Vascular strip

The external surface of the tympanic membrane is supplied by the deep auricular branch of the maxillary artery. This artery provides a leash of prominent vessels that pass down the superior canal wall. This area is called the 'vascular strip'. (Left ear)

Figure 1.75
Collapsing external auditory canal

In some patients a structural deficiency in the surrounding and supporting fibroelastic cartilage allows the external portion of the auditory canal to collapse, leaving only a slit-like narrow lumen. Pressure against such an external auditory canal from a headphone may increase the amount of collapse to such an extent that the external canal becomes completely occluded. (Right ear)

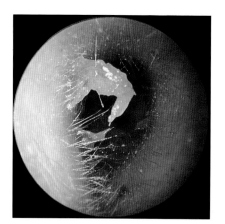

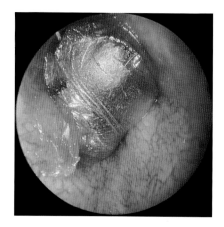

Figure 1.76
Cerumen

The openings of the ceruminous glands are located near the base of the hairs of the cartilaginous canal. The ceruminous glands produce a clear colourless secretion. Whilst the secretions of the ceruminous glands are called 'cerumen', by tradition, this term is most commonly used to refer to earwax (see Figure 1.78). The normal outward migration of the epithelium lining the deep meatus will normally carry keratin debris and cerumen out into the cartilaginous portion of the external auditory canal. In this patient a small collection of soft, light-brown cerumen is seen being elevated by the hairs of the cartilaginous canal. (Right ear)

Figure 1.77
Veil of cerumen

In this patient the superficial area of outwardly migrating keratin has become flipped across the external auditory canal where it lies like a drape or veil. This appearance most commonly results from the use of cotton–tipped applicators, which elevate and rotate the superficial layer of the keratin lining the external auditory canal. (Right ear)

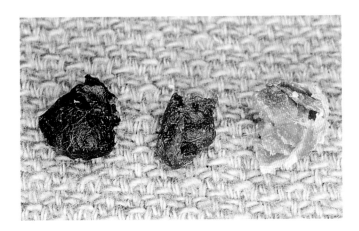

Figure 1.78
Colours of cerumen

Cerumen or earwax is a complex mixture of desquamated keratin
squames and hairs, combined with the secretions of the sebaceous
and ceruminous glands. Cerumen varies in colour from golden yellow
through brown to black.

Figure 1.79
Colour of cerumen

The pigment(s) responsible for the coloration of cerumen has yet to be
identified. Burnt ochre is the most common colour of cerumen, as
seen in this smear made from a piece of dark-brown cerumen.

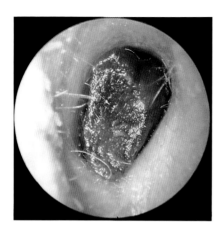

Figure 1.80
Cerumen accumulation

While cerumen is normally removed from the external auditory canal by the process of epithelial migration, in some patients it gradually collects along the floor of the external auditory canal. Cerumen may accumulate to such an extent that it totally occludes the lumen of the external auditory canal. (Right ear)

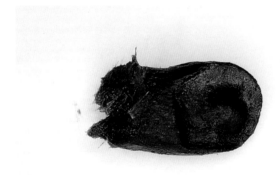

Figure 1.81
Cerumen accumulation

In some patients the plug of cerumen may accumulate to such an extent that it totally fills the external auditory canal and produces a mould or cast of the canal. Note the impression of the lateral surface of the tympanic membrane on the right side of this extensive cerumen plug.

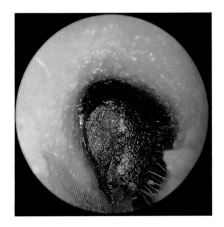

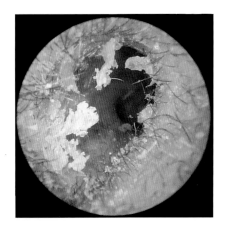

Figure 1.82
Inspissated hard cerumen

The external canal of this patient (left ear) is plugged with a bony-hard accumulation of cerumen. Black cerumen is more commonly encountered in the older age groups, and when it becomes dry and inspissated in consistency, it is more difficult to remove.

Figure 1.83
Oriental wax

Cerumen occurs in two forms: wet and dry. The usual type of cerumen found in Orientals is the dry type, commonly referred to as 'rice bran' wax, as it resembles particles of rice bran.

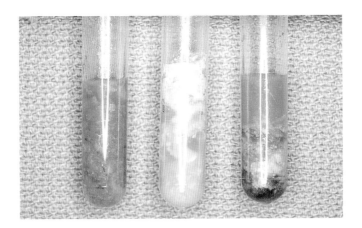

Figure 1.84
Effective ceruminolytics

Ceruminolytics are compounds that soften and liquefy earwax. The most effective ceruminolytics have an aqueous base. Note the swelling and dissolution of a cerumen plug caused by these aqueous solutions (from the left: sodium bicarbonate, hydrogen peroxide and distilled water).

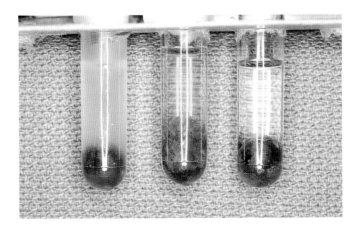

Figure 1.85
Ineffective ceruminolytics

In contrast, oily based solutions are not effective in breaking up a cerumen plug as seen in these organic solutions (from the left: Cerumol, Cerumenex and olive oil).

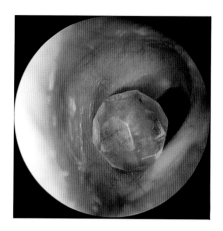

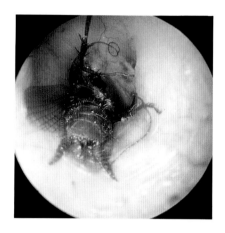

Figure 1.86
Foreign body

A wide variety of foreign bodies may become lodged in the external auditory canal whether by accident, neglect or deliberate insertion. The signs and symptoms of a foreign body depend on its size, location and composition of material. A purple plastic bead was inserted into the external auditory canal in this young child. A general anaesthetic was required for safe removal owing to the child's lack of cooperation. (Right ear)

Figure 1.87
Foreign body

Animate foreign bodies, such as this large cockroach, may produce objective tinnitus, itching and severe pain. Injury to the epithelium from the sharp spurs on the insect's hind legs produced an acute otitis externa. It was not until the otitis externa had been treated successfully with topical antibiotics that the primary cause was observed.

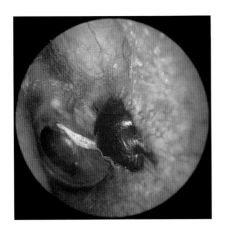

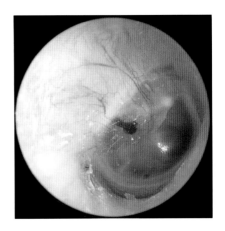

Figure 1.88
Haematoma, external auditory canal

The epithelium lining the bony or
deep canal is extremely thin and
easily traumatized. The use of a
cotton-tipped applicator in aural
cleansing can easily produce a
haematoma in the skin overlying the
floor of the bony external auditory
canal. Following débridement of the
external auditory canal, a more
extensive subepithelial haematoma
has formed, which has elevated the
superficial keratin layer. (Left ear)

Figure 1.89
Haematoma, tympanic membrane

This asymptomatic haematoma
located just behind the handle of the
malleus resulted from the deep
insertion of a cotton-tipped applicator
during aural toilet. The friction of the
cotton bud has produced a small
superficial haematoma of the
epithelium covering the tympanic
membrane. (Right ear)

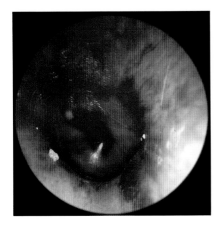

Figure 1.90
Haematoma, tympanic membrane

Following relatively traumatic wax
curettage, a large haematoma has
developed over the deep portion of
the bony external auditory canal. The
haematoma has tracked down in the
loose subcutaneous tissue on either
side of the handle of the malleus.
(Left ear)

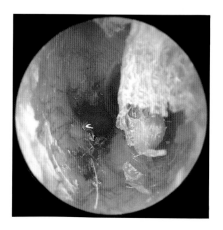

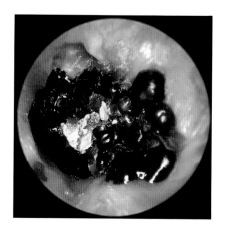

Figure 1.91
Laceration, external auditory canal

The thin and delicate skin lining the bony external auditory canal has been lacerated during wax curettage. Active bleeding through the laceration can be seen. Because of the vascularity of the skin in this area, such bleeding may be troublesome and if not stopped may fill the deep canal with blood.

Figure 1.92
Old blood clot in external auditory canal

A blood clot in the external auditory canal should be removed when it is relatively fresh and still soft and jelly–like in consistency. If clotted blood is allowed to remain in the external auditory canal, it will gradually become converted into a bony-hard, black, tar-like mixture, which is extremely difficult to remove.

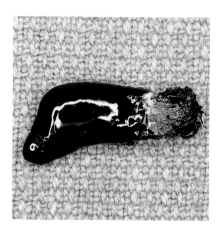

Figure 1.93
Blood clot in external auditory canal

Bleeding from a traumatic laceration of an external auditory canal allowed this clot to fill the external auditory canal. Note how the outer (right) side of the clot has undergone desiccation and hardening while the deeper (left) portion of the clot still has a jelly-like consistency.

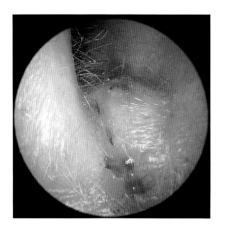

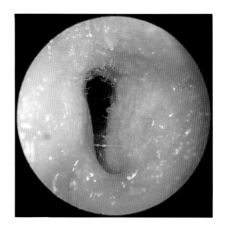

Figure 1.94
Acute localized otitis externa (furuncle)

A furuncle is a small staphylococcal abscess that arises at the base of a hair follicle. Furuncles only occur in the outer cartilaginous hair-bearing portion of the external canal. They present as a red and extremely painful localized swelling.

Figure 1.95
Acute otitis externa

Acute diffuse otitis externa ('swimmer's ear') is the most common infection of the external ear canal. The most common predisposing factors are exposure to moisture and local trauma. *Pseudomonas aeruginosa* is the usual pathogen. Initially the skin lining the external auditory canal becomes oedematous and has a shiny appearance, with extreme tenderness; as the infection progresses, the swelling of the epithelial lining of the external canal increases and the infected epithelium exudes a watery or serous discharge. (Right ear)

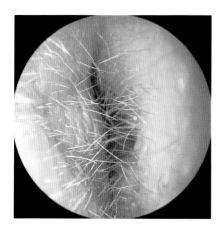

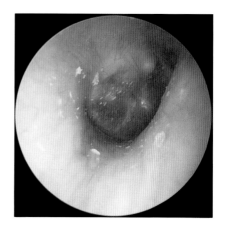

Figure 1.96
Severe acute otitis externa

As the acute otitis externa
progresses, the swelling of the
epithelium lining of the external
canal may increase to such an extent
that the lumen is totally occluded.
Severe local pain and trismus are
usually present. (Right ear)

Figure 1.97
Chronic otitis externa

Chronic otitis externa, in contrast
with acute otitis externa, is usually a
painless condition in which itching,
irritation and scanty otorrhoea are
the predominant symptoms. The skin
of the external auditory canal is
thickened, shiny and usually
erythematous. Normal cerumen is
usually absent, as seen in this
patient. (Right ear)

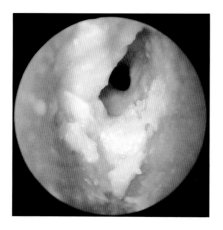

Figure 1.98
Chronic otitis externa

Chronic otitis externa may be the
result of a bacterial, fungal or mixed
infection. In this patient, the deep
meatus is filled with a collection of
moist, macerated keratin squames.
(Right ear)

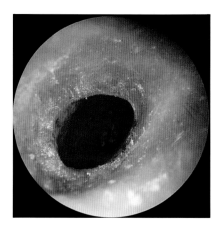

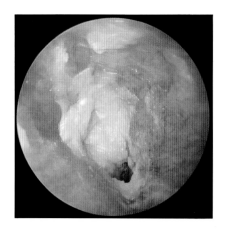

Figure 1.99
Acquired stenosis of external auditory canal

In this patient chronic trauma to the epithelium lining the bony canal and an associated chronic otitis externa have produced an acquired stricture and stenosis of the deep external auditory canal. The tiny pinhole-sized lumen that remains is, however, sufficient for normal hearing as long as the lumen is kept free of debris. (Right ear)

Figure 1.100
Otomycosis due to *Candida albicans*

Infection of the external auditory canal by fungal organisms is called 'otomycosis'. The most common pathogenic fungi involved are *Aspergillus* and *Candida* spp. Infections with *Candida albicans* do not show any morphological evidence of fungi and as a result the diagnosis of otomycosis in these patients can only be made by culture. Patients with candidal otitis externa frequently present with a creamy-white exudate within the deep canal, as seen in this patient. (Left ear)

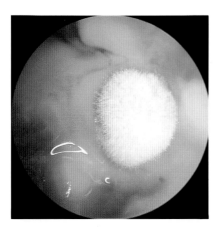

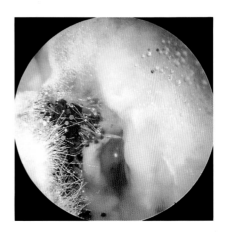

Figure 1.101
Otomycosis due to *Aspergillus niger*

Otomycosis caused by *Aspergillus* can usually be diagnosed by the presence of a white, fluffy, cotton-like material, which represents the fungal hyphae. (Left ear)

Figure 1.102
Otomycosis due to *Aspergillus niger*

Another diagnostic feature of *Aspergillus* infections is the presence of small coloured particles (conidiophores). Note the collection of black debris and the fungal hyphae in this patient with otomycosis due to *Aspergillus niger*. (Right ear)

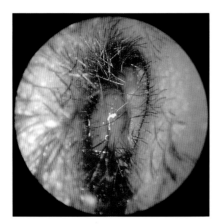

Figure 1.103
Malignant otitis externa

Malignant otitis externa is a severe and locally aggressive form of otitis externa that occurs in elderly diabetics and immunocompromised patients. The causative organism is usually *Pseudomonas aeruginosa*. Classically, malignant otitis externa presents as a severe pain in the ear associated with the appearance of exuberant granulation tissue arising from the floor of the external auditory canal at the junction of the bony and cartilaginous portions. (Right ear)

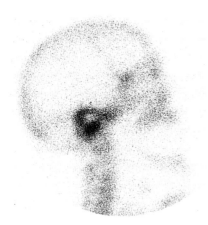

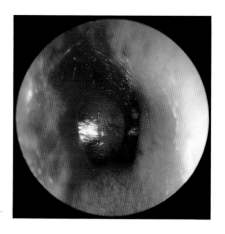

Figure 1.104
Malignant otitis externa:
gallium scan

The spreading infection of malignant
otitis externa can be seen in this
gallium scan. (Right ear)

Figure 1.105
Myringitis bullosa (bullous
myringitis)

Bullous myringitis is a specific form
of viral otitis externa characterized by
the appearance of blebs on the
tympanic membrane and in the skin
of the deep bony meatus, and
associated with severe local pain. The
bleb seen on the posterior bony canal
wall and adjacent tympanic
membrane contains a serosanguinous
effusion. Note the small collection of
blood in the more dependent portion
of the bulla. (Right ear)

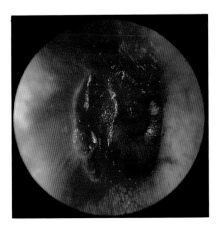

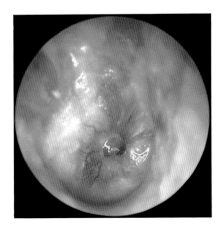

Figure 1.106
Severe myringitis bullosa (bullous myringitis)

Following rupture and aspiration of the contents of the large bulla seen in Figure 1.105, the true extent of the subcutaneous and intracutaneous haemorrhage can be seen. Note the extensive haemorrhage along the handle of the malleus. (Right ear)

Figure 1.107
Localized granular myringitis

A chronic infection of the tympanic membrane associated with the appearance and persistence of painless, bright-red granulation tissue is termed 'granular myringitis'. Granular myringitis appears to be the result of chronic superficial infection of the thin epithelium covering the lateral surface of the tympanic membrane. Granular myringitis occurs in two distinct varieties: localized granulation tissue and diffuse granulation tissue. The pathogens responsible for granular myringitis may be either bacterial or fungal. In this patient the chronic inflammation was the result of a candidal infection. (Right ear)

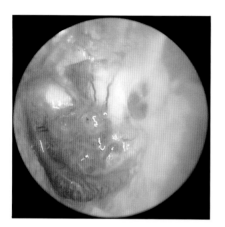

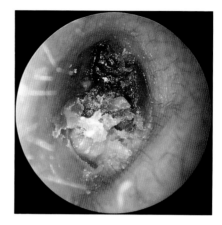

Figure 1.108
Diffuse granular myringitis

In this patient a large portion of the
tympanic membrane surface is
covered with a diffuse granulation
tissue. (Left ear)

Figure 1.109
Keratosis obturans

Keratosis obturans is a condition in
which the external auditory canal
becomes occluded by an
accumulation of keratin squamous
debris. This condition appears to be
the result of a defect in the normal
self-cleansing migratory mechanism
of the external auditory canal which
allows the normally removed
desquamated superficial keratin
squames to accumulate in the
external canal. (Right ear)

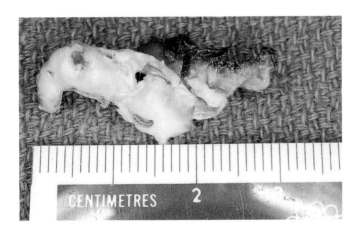

Figure 1.110
Keratin plug

The typical white plug which had occluded the external auditory canal
is seen here. The lateral surface of the plug is covered with what
appears to be relatively normal cerumen.

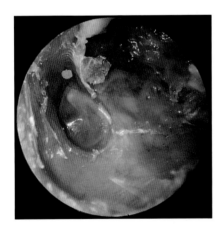

Figure 1.111
**Automastoidectomy secondary to
keratosis obturans**

The slowly enlarging plug of keratin
squamous debris may exert enough
pressure on the bone of the deep
canal to cause substantial
reabsorption. In these patients,
following removal of the plug, an
extremely wide, scooped-out external
canal may be seen. In this patient
the persistence of a keratin plug
within the external auditory canal for
a period of 5 years caused such
pressure that the entire posterior
bony canal wall and mastoid wall
were resorbed, resulting in an
automastoidectomy. (Left ear)

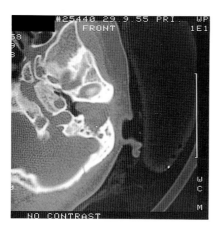

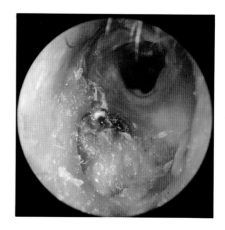

Figure 1.112
Automastoidectomy secondary to keratosis obturans

The massive keratin plug can be clearly seen in this axial CT scan. Note how the plug has caused total resorption of the posterior bony canal wall and erosion of the mastoid process. (Left ear)

Figure 1.113
Osteitis of tympanic bone (cholesteatoma of external auditory canal)

Osteitis of the external auditory canal appears to result from local trauma disrupting the thin epithelium and underlying periosteum that overlies the tympanic bone. This allows the exposed tympanic bone to become infected, with the development of chronic osteitis. This results in an ulceration of the skin lining the floor of the external auditory canal and exposure of devitalized bone. (Right ear)

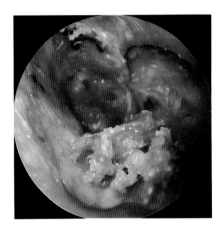

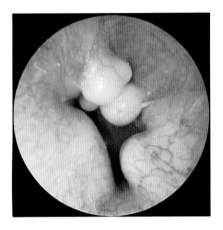

Figure 1.114
Irradiation osteitis

High levels of radiation may cause
osteoradionecrosis of the tympanic
bone with ulceration and
sequestration similar to that seen in
benign osteitis of tympanic bone.
(Left ear)

Figure 1.115
Multiple exostoses

Exostoses of the bony ear canal,
localized areas of benign bony
hypertrophy, are usually multiple.
They are thought to result from
stimulation of the periosteum
covering the medial surface of the
tympanic bone by cold temperatures,
e.g. swimming in cold water. The
white colour of the exostoses is the
result of thinning of the epithelium
over the exostoses, allowing the ivory
white colour of the underlying bone
to be seen. In this patient the
external canal has been significantly
narrowed by multiple exostoses;
nevertheless, the lumen is still of
sufficient calibre for normal sound
conduction and epithelial migration.
(Left ear)

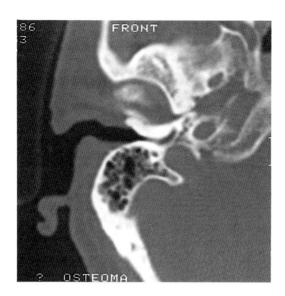

Figure 1.116
Multiple exostoses: CT scan

The dense ivory bone of exostoses arising from
the anterior surface of the tympanic bone can
be seen in this axial high-resolution CT scan.
(Courtesy of Dr L Shankar.)

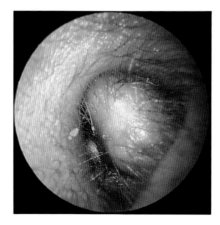

Figure 1.117
Osteoma of tympanic bone

Osteomas of the deep ear
canal are benign bony
tumours that are relatively
uncommon and usually
solitary in occurrence.
Osteomas appear as bony-
hard pedunculated or
sessile masses covered by
normal canal skin. The
large bony mass arising
from this anterior canal
wall was a pedunculated
solitary osteoma.

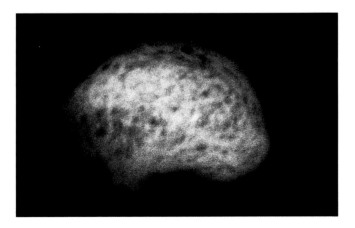

Figure 1.118
Osteoma of tympanic bone: dental radiograph

Unlike exostoses, osteomas consist of a spongy or cancellous type of
bone, as can be seen in this dental radiograph of a surgically removed
osteoma.

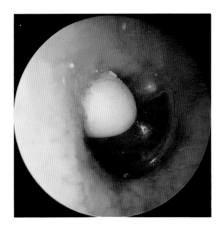

Figure 1.119
Epidermal inclusion cysts

Epidermal inclusion cysts
in the skin of the external
auditory canal usually
result from trauma with
implantation of epidermal
cells into the dermis of the
deep canal epithelium.
Epidermal inclusion cysts
have a pearly white
coloration and are soft to
palpation. The epidermal
inclusion cyst seen in the
10 o'clock position in this
patient developed in the
site of an endomeatal
incision undertaken for
access to the middle ear for
stapedectomy. (Right ear)

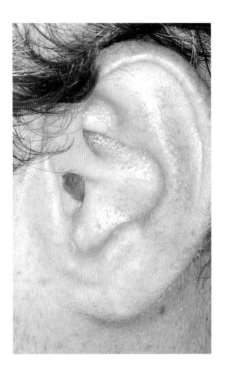

Figure 1.120
Aural polyp

An aural polyp protruding from the external auditory meatus may arise from the canal skin or from the mucosa of the middle ear passing through a perforation in the tympanic membrane. Careful assessment of such aural polyps is required to identify the origin prior to excision. Topical steroids are nearly always a helpful initial treatment.

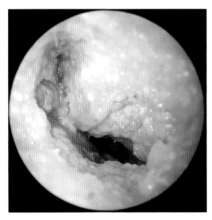

Figure 1.121
Carcinoma of external auditory canal

Any unusual and persistent lesion arising from the skin of the external auditory canal should be carefully investigated and biopsied. This knobbly lesion was a squamous cell carcinoma. (Left ear)

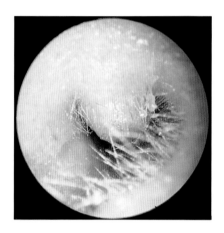

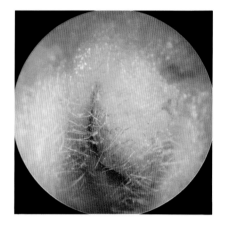

Figure 1.122
Adenocarcinoma of external auditory canal

This innocuous dome-shaped subcutaneous mass was diagnosed by excisional biopsy as an adenoid cystic adenocarcinoma. (Left ear)

Figure 1.123
Ceruminoma of external auditory canal

In contrast, this large subcutaneous lesion arising from the left anterior canal wall and narrowing the lumen of the external canal was a ceruminoma. These locally aggressive tumours arise in the cartilaginous portion of the external auditory canal from ceruminous gland tissue.

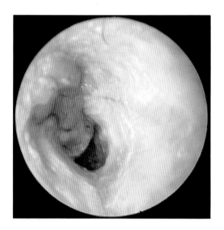

Figure 1.124
Secondary adenocystic adenocarcinoma of external auditory canal

The irregular pink subcutaneous mass invading the skin lining the deep anterior canal wall of this left ear is an adenoid cystic adenocarcinoma, which has spread posteriorly from the parotid gland.

Middle ear

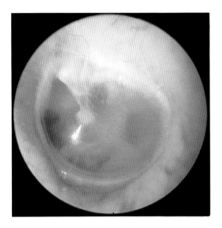

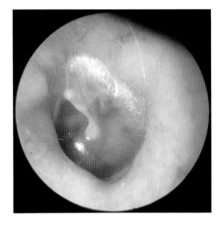

Figure 1.125
Normal right tympanic membrane

The normal tympanic membrane is a pale-grey, ovoid, semi-transparent membrane, which sits at the medial end of the bony external auditory canal. The tympanic membrane acts like a semi-transparent window through which the middle ear and some of its contents may frequently be visualized. Note in this photograph the handle of the malleus with its short process superiorly and its cone of light antcroinferiorly. The long process of the incus can be seen in the posterosuperior quadrant, as can the chorda tympani nerve. (Left ear)

Figure 1.126
Prominent pars flaccida

The upper one–fifth of the tympanic membrane, the pars flaccida, has a thin and mobile fibrous middle layer. The pars flaccida of this normal left tympanic membrane is very well developed. Note the slight outward bulging of the pars flaccida at the level of the head of the malleus.

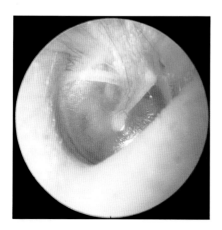

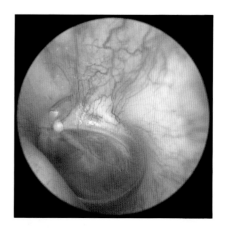

Figure 1.127
Chorda tympani nerve

A very prominent chorda tympani nerve can been seen passing across the posterosuperior quadrant of this right tympanic membrane. Note the prominent posterior bulging of the anteroinferior bony canal wall, which hides the anterior sulcus of the tympanic membrane. (Left ear)

Figure 1.128
Vascular strip

The lateral surface of the tympanic membrane is supplied by the deep auricular branch of the maxillary artery, which sends a leash of prominent vessels down the superior canal wall. This area is called the 'vascular strip'. (Left ear)

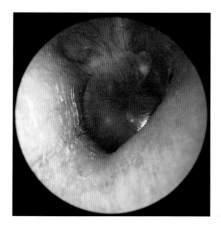

Figure 1.129
Prominent tympanic membrane vasculature

In some patients the blood supply of the vascular strip along the superior portion of the deep external auditory canal and the vessels that run from the vascular strip down either side of the handle of the malleus are unduly prominent. This is a variation of normal, which should not be interpreted as providing evidence of inflammation, i.e. an early acute otitis media. (Right ear)

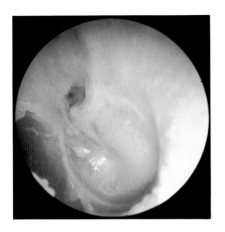

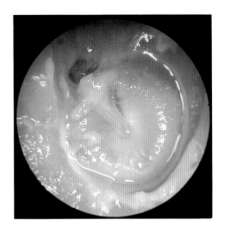

Figure 1.130
Apparent shape of tympanic
membrane

The tympanic membrane is located
obliquely to the central axis of the
external auditory canal. This oblique
angulation gives the examiner a false
impression that the tympanic
membrane is flat and oval in shape,
as seen in this cadaveric specimen
photographed through the external
auditory canal. (Left ear)

Figure 1.131
Actual shape of tympanic
membrane

In reality, the shape of the tympanic
membrane is essentially circular and
conical, as seen in this photograph of
the previous specimen taken through
a hole in the mastoid drilled at right
angles to the actual axis of the
tympanic membrane. (Left ear)

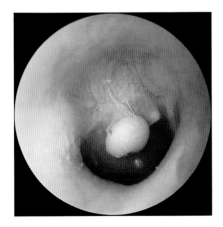

Figure 1.132
Congenital epidermal inclusion
cyst of tympanic membrane

The white cystic structure located in
the central portion of the tympanic
membrane is a benign congenital
epidermal cyst located lateral to the
fibrous middle layer of the tympanic
membrane. (Right ear)

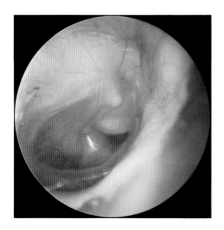

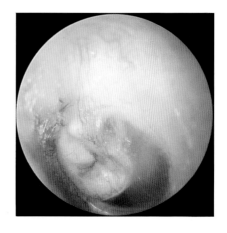

Figure 1.133
Small congenital epidermal cholesteatoma

The white cystic structure seen just behind the tympanic membrane in the anterosuperior quadrant is a typical small congenital epidermal cholesteatoma. (Right ear)

Figure 1.134
Medium-sized congenital epidermal cholesteatoma

The large white cystic structure seen deep to the tympanic membrane in this middle ear is a medium-sized congenital epidermoid cholesteatoma. (Left ear)

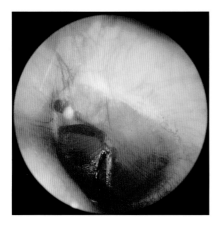

Figure 1.135
Traumatic perforation

Traumatic perforations of the tympanic membrane are the result of either sudden changes in pressure in the external auditory canal or direct trauma from an object inserted through the external auditory canal and into the tympanic membrane. The traumatic perforation seen in the anteroinferior quadrant of this young boy's tympanic membrane resulted from indirect trauma—a slap on the ear by his irate schoolmaster. (Left ear)

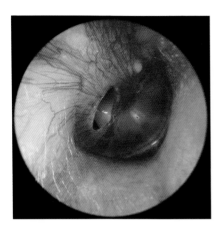

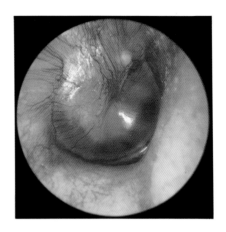

Figure 1.136
Traumatic perforation

The large linear perforation over the
incudostapedial joint in the
posterosuperior quadrant of this
patient's tympanic membrane
resulted from direct trauma—the
insertion of a cotton-tipped applicator
too deeply into the external auditory
canal. (Right ear)

Figure 1.137
Healed traumatic perforation

Six weeks later the perforation seen
in Figure 1.136 had healed
completely with no visible sequel. If
kept clean and dry, most traumatic
perforations will heal spontaneously
within 2 months.

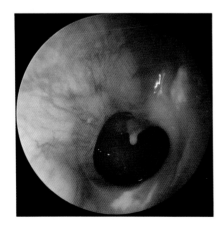

Figure 1.138
**Thermal burn injury of tympanic
membrane**

The tympanic membrane may be
perforated by welding sparks or hot
liquids that are inadvertently poured
down the external auditory canal. The
large subtotal perforation in this
tympanic membrane resulted from an
accidental spill of hot grease down the
external auditory canal. (Right ear)

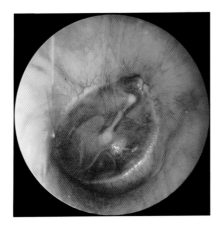

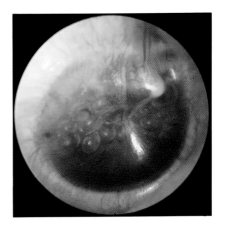

Figure 1.139
Barotrauma

The inability to equalize intratympanic with atmospheric pressure during descent in an aircraft or while diving in water may cause barotraumatic damage of the tympanic membrane or middle ear. This patient shows the classic appearance of barotrauma following flying (6 hours earlier): there is a subepithelial haemorrhage along the handle of the malleus and over the posterosuperior annulus, with strands of golden-yellow fluid behind the lower half of the tympanic membrane. (Right ear)

Figure 1.140
Barotrauma

This patient developed a dark-orange serous effusion following barotrauma caused by travelling in an aircraft while having an upper respiratory infection. (Right ear)

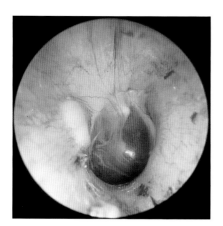

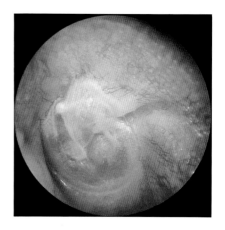

Figure 1.141
Temporal bone fracture

Temporal bone fractures may extend into the bony external auditory canal leaving telltale raised subepithelial bony fragments or subepithelial clefts along the fracture line. Note the displaced chip of bone beneath the epithelium of the posterior bony external canal in the 9 o'clock position. (Right ear)

Figure 1.142
Temporal bone fracture

Note the diastasis of the posterosuperior bony canal wall in the 3 o'clock position. (Right ear)

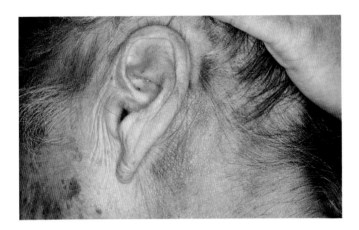

Figure 1.143
Battle's sign

Temporal bone fractures may be associated with bruising of the skin over the mastoid process, as seen in this patient. This is referred to as 'Battle's sign'.

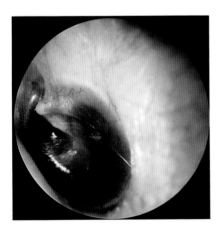

Figure 1.144

The presence of extravasated blood or blood-stained fluid in the middle ear is called a 'haemotympanum'. A haemotympanum may develop following head injury with temporal bone fracture, following barotrauma or in association with a severe otitis media. The presence of blood within the middle ear causes the tympanic membrane to appear deeply coloured, with the colour ranging from dark red to gun–metal grey. The older, dark-brown bloody fluid in this middle ear has coloured the tympanic membrane black. (Left ear)

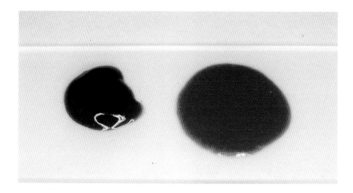

Figure 1.145
Haemotympanum fluid

The colour of fluid in the ear of a patient with a haemotympanum may vary from bright red, as seen on the right, to a chocolate-brown colour, as seen on the left.

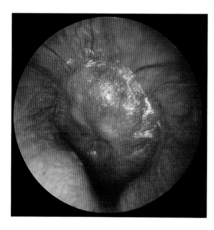

Figure 1.146
Early acute otitis media:
stage of redness

The earliest changes in acute suppurative otitis media consist of redness, oedema and swelling in the pars flaccida (the upper fifth of the tympanic membrane). In this patient the pars flaccida shows increased redness, oedema and marked outward bulging. (Left ear)

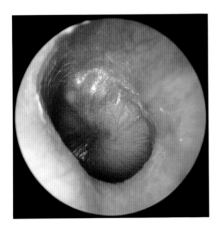

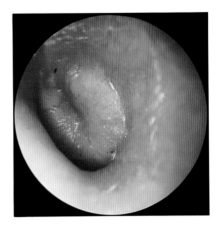

Figure 1.147
Otitis media: stage of suppuration

The stage of redness is shortly followed (24–48 hours) by the development of a mucopurulent exudate within the middle ear cleft. This creamy-white fluid rapidly fills the middle ear and causes the tympanic membrane gradually to bulge outwards. (Left ear)

Figure 1.148
Severe acute otitis media

In this patient the middle ear cleft is filled with creamy-white mucopurulent material under pressure, which has caused the tympanic membrane to bulge laterally. (Left ear)

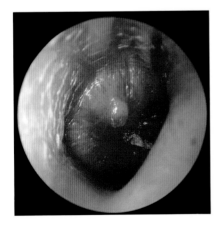

Figure 1.149
Severe acute otitis media

The small outward bulge in the centre of this tympanic membrane is an area in which the fibrous middle layer has become necrotic and the thin epithelium is being herniated laterally by the pressure of the purulent fluid within the middle ear. It is through this area that a tiny perforation will shortly develop to allow the infected material within the middle ear to drain into the external auditory canal, acting like a 'spontaneous' myringotomy. (Right ear)

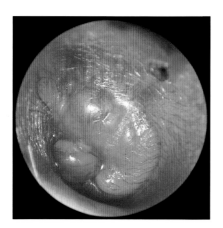

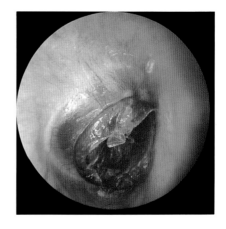

Figure 1.150
Severe acute otitis media

In this patient the entire tympanic membrane is bulging laterally under the pressure of the infected purulent debris in the middle ear. (Left ear)

Figure 1.151
Serous and keratin casts of the tympanic membrane

In some cases of severe otitis media the infection may spread right through the tympanic membrane to such an extent that serous fluid weeps from the lateral surface of the tympanic membrane. The inflamed squamous epithelium covering the tympanic membrane produces keratin squames at an increased rate. The end result is a golden-yellow brittle 'cast' covering the surface of the tympanic membrane. (Left ear)

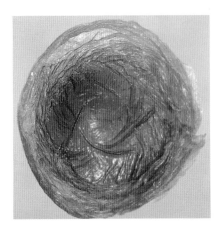

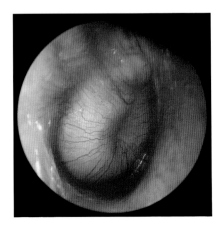

Figure 1.152
Serous and keratin cast of
tympanic membrane

Over time, following resolution of the infection, the cast covering the tympanic membrane will slowly separate and be carried out along the external auditory canal by normal migration. Initially this circular cast had covered the entire tympanic membrane; it was retrieved from the external canal of a young child.

Figure 1.153
Mastoiditis

An incompletely treated or prolonged acute suppurative otitis media may extend from the middle ear into the mastoid air cell system, producing an acute mastoiditis. In this patient the tympanic membrane is bulging out because of the presence of a chronic accumulation of purulent debris within the middle ear. (Right ear)

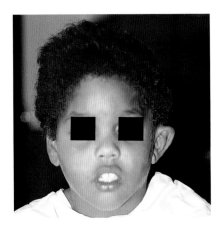

Figure 1.154
Subperiosteal abscess

A collection of pus under pressure beneath the periosteum over the left mastoid cortex will elevate the pinna, producing an outstanding ear, as seen in this patient.

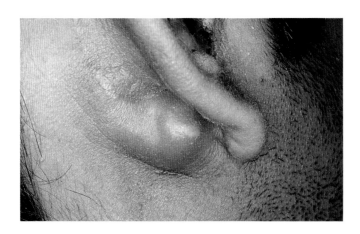

Figure 1.155
Subperiosteal abscess

In this patient the infection within the mastoid has perforated through the cortex laterally to produce a subcutaneous abscess over the mastoid tip. A large cholesteatoma was the predisposing factor.

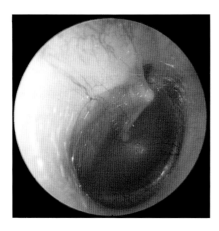

Figure 1.156
Mucoid otitis media

Mucoid otitis media is the most common cause of hearing loss in childhood. The mucoid fluid is opalescent in colour, and consequently one cannot view through the tympanic membrane into the middle ear. The structures of the middle ear are obscured by this opalescent yellowish fluid. (Right ear)

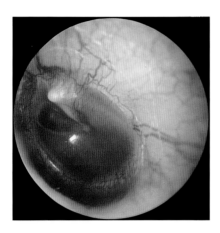

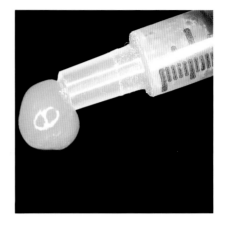

Figure 1.157
Mucoid otitis media

The mucoid fluid in this middle ear has an orange tinge. Note the tiny air bubble anterior to the malleus handle. (Left ear)

Figure 1.158
Mucoid otitis media

This fluid removed at myringotomy shows characteristic coloration and opacification of the middle ear exudate seen in patients with mucoid otitis media. Note the yellowish discolouration and thick tenacity.

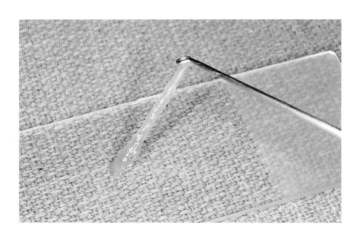

Figure 1.159
Mucoid otitis media

In this patient the fluid removed from the middle ear is opalescent and rubbery in consistency.

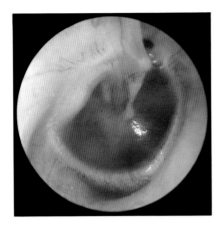

Figure 1.160
Serous otitis media

Serous otitis media results from persistent and complete eustachian tube obstruction. This condition is characterized by the accumulation of a clear, golden-yellow or straw-coloured, thin, uninfected, watery serous fluid within the middle ear. The tympanic membrane shows a yellowish discolouration from the fluid within. (Right ear)

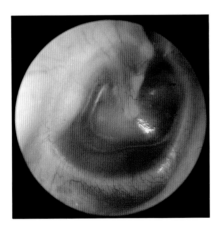

Figure 1.161
Serous otitis media post-Valsalva

This is the same patient as shown in Figure 1.160 following autoinflation by means of the Valsalva manœuvre (attempting to exhale through the nose against pinched nostrils), which forces air up the eustachian tube, reventilating the middle ear, as seen here. Note how most of the golden-yellow watery fluid within the middle ear has been displaced by air. (Right ear)

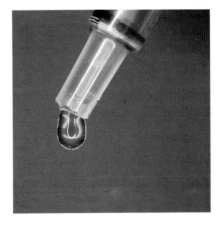

Figure 1.162
Serous fluid

The fluid obtained at myringotomy from patients with serous otitis media is clear, yellow or straw-coloured and watery in consistency. The colour of the fluid within the middle ear gives the tympanic membrane a yellowish colour.

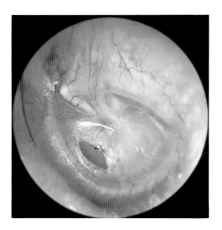

Figure 1.163
Myringotomy

Note the anteroinferior myringotomy
incision through which fluid in the
middle ear has been aspirated. The
myringotomy incision usually heals
spontaneously within 7–14 days.
Following removal of the fluid, the
true colour of the tympanic
membrane can be seen. (Left ear)

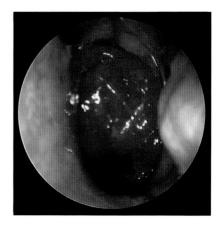

Figure 1.164
Carcinoma of the nasopharynx

A carcinoma of the nasopharynx
must be suspected in any adult
patient who presents with a
persistent serous otitis media. In this
patient the carcinoma arising from
the posterior wall of the left
nasopharynx was discovered with a
Hopkins rod nasopharyngeal
endoscopic examination.

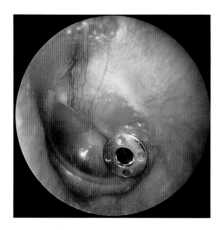

Figure 1.165
Ventilation tube

Ventilation tubes allow more
permanent aeration, ventilation and
drainage of the middle ear. Note the
stainless steel Reuter bobbin present
in this patient's left tympanic
membrane. (Left ear)

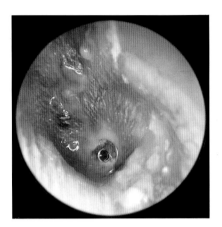

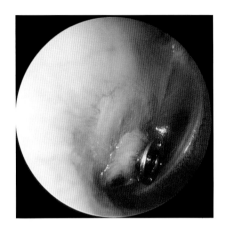

Figure 1.166
Otitis media in a patient with a ventilation tube

This patient with a ventilation tube in place developed an otitis media. The external auditory canal is filled with a mixture of air bubbles and purulent fluid, which has drained into the external auditory canal through the lumen of the tube. (Right ear)

Figure 1.167
Extruding ventilation tube

Most ventilation tubes spontaneously extrude from 3 months to 2 years following insertion. The time interval between insertion and extrusion is a function of the individual patient and the type of tube inserted. Note the tiny collar of keratin accumulating behind the outer flange of this stainless steel Reuter bobbin tube. The action of the tympanic membrane and its accumulating collar of keratin has almost completely lifted the bobbin out of its insertion site in the tympanic membrane. (Right ear)

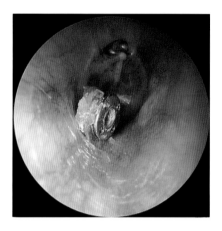

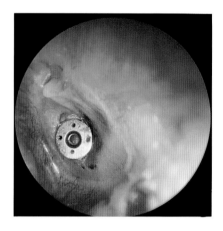

Figure 1.168
Extruded tube

Once a tube has extruded from the tympanic membrane, it will be carried outward by the normal migration of the epithelium lining the deep external auditory canal. (Right ear)

Figure 1.169
Blocked ventilation tube

The lumen of a ventilation tube must remain patent if the tube is to perform its intended functions: aeration, pressure equalization and, when necessary, drainage. The lumen of this stainless steel Reuter bobbin has become blocked by a small amount of clotted blood. (Left ear)

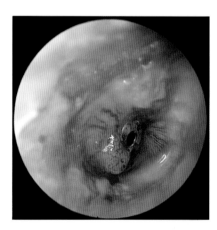

Figure 1.170
Tube granuloma

In approximately 1% of cases, the keratin collar that accumulates around a ventilation tube inserted in the tympanic membrane will incite a foreign body granulomatous reaction. This results in the local production of an exuberant mass of granulation tissue. The vascular lesion arising from the surface of the tympanic membrane and covering the inferior portion of the stainless steel ventilation tube is a tube granuloma. (Right ear)

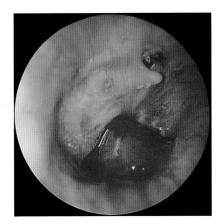

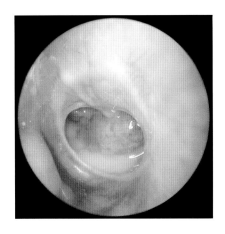

Figure 1.171
Tube granuloma

The larger polypoid granuloma present in this tympanic membrane completely engulfed the stainless steel Reuter bobbin ventilation tube that had previously been inserted into the tympanic membrane. (Right ear)

Figure 1.172
Chronic suppurative otitis media

Chronic suppurative otitis media is characterized by a painless persistent otorrhoea and a perforation in the tympanic membrane. This patient with a large central perforation has developed an acute viral upper respiratory infection. The mucosa lining the middle ear has become infected and as a result has produced a creamy-white, thick mucoid fluid. (Left ear)

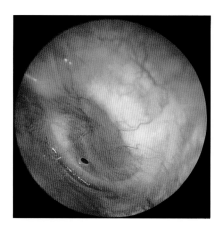

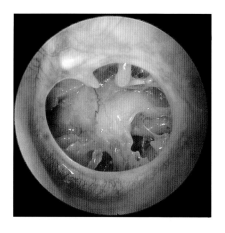

Figure 1.173
Pinpoint central perforation

This patient has a small pinpoint perforation, which developed following an episode of acute otitis media. (Left ear)

Figure 1.174
Total perforation of the tympanic membrane

In this patient there is a total perforation of the tympanic membrane. Note how most of the handle of the malleus is missing. (Left ear)

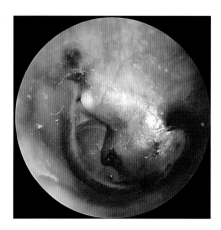

Figure 1.175
Cholesterol granuloma

This yellow-brown mass within the middle ear, which is pushing the tympanic membrane laterally, is a small cholesterol foreign body granuloma. (Left ear)

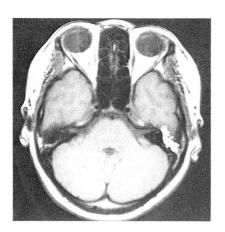

Figure 1.176
Cholesterol granuloma: MRI scan

The cholesterol crystals within a
cholesterol granuloma are illuminated
on an MRI scan; as a result a
cholesterol granuloma is easily
diagnosed with MRI.

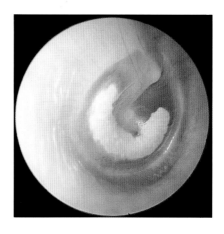

Figure 1.177
Tympanosclerosis

Tympanosclerotic plaques consist of
collections of thickened hyalinized
collagen located in the fibrous middle
layer of the tympanic membrane.
Tympanosclerotic plaques result from
previous middle ear infections. In
this patient the tympanic membrane
contains one large horseshoe-shaped
tympanosclerotic plaque curving
around the lower portion of the
malleus. (Right ear)

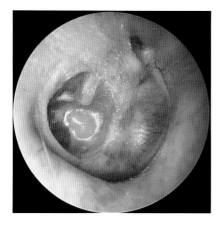

Figure 1.178
Retracted tympanic membrane

In this patient, because of chronic
negative pressure within the middle
ear, the posterior superior quadrant
of the tympanic membrane has
become retracted medially. Note how
it is draped over the long process of
the incus and also over the
promontory. (Right ear)

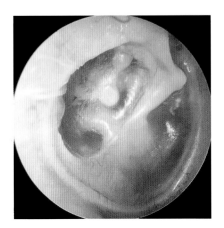

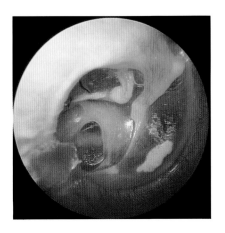

Figure 1.179
Myringostapediopexy

In this patient, as the result of chronic negative pressure, the tympanic membrane has become retracted over its posterior half. The lenticular process of the incus has eroded and the head of the stapes can be seen directly in contact with the tympanic membrane. This situation is known as a 'myringostapediopexy'.

Figure 1.180
Self-cleansing retraction pocket

Chronic intratympanic negative pressure may cause the tympanic membrane to become retracted and thinned, forming a 'retraction pocket'. Retraction pockets occur most commonly in the posterior half of the tympanic membrane. So long as retraction pockets are self-cleansing they do not appear to be at risk for the development of a cholesteatoma. (Right ear)

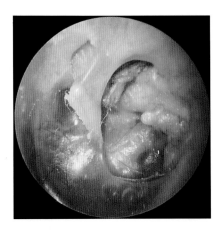

Figure 1.181
Non-self-cleansing retraction pocket

When the epithelium lining the retraction pocket loses its normal migratory abilities and consequently is no longer self-cleansing, keratin may accumulate within the retraction pocket. These patients are at risk for the development of a cholesteatoma in this area. (Left ear)

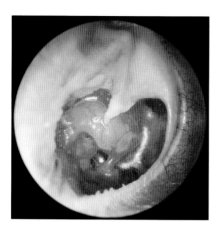

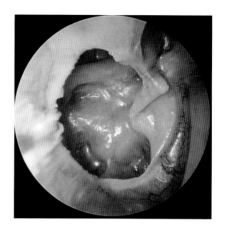

Figure 1.182
Middle ear atelectasis

Long-standing negative intratympanic pressure may cause almost complete resorption of the fibrous middle layer of the tympanic membrane. The result is an extensive retraction pocket, which may appear on first glance to be a large central perforation. (Right ear)

Figure 1.183
Adhesive otitis media

The last and most severe stage in the effect of chronic negative pressure on the middle ear is a condition known as 'adhesive otitis media': the medial surface of the tympanic membrane has become attached by adhesions to the medial wall of the middle ear. This is generally an irreversible condition. (Right ear)

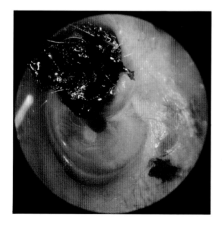

Figure 1.184
Attic cholesteatoma

Crusts overlying the attic frequently hide significant pathology and especially a cholesteatoma. (Left ear)

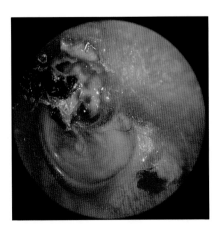

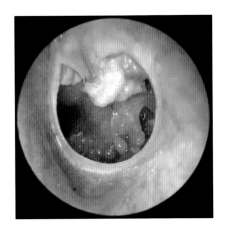

Figure 1.185
Attic cholesteatoma

This is the same patient as in Figure 1.184 following removal of the blood-stained serous crust. Note the collection of keratin debris arising from an attic cholesteatoma. (Left ear)

Figure 1.186
Middle ear cholesteatoma

In this patient a cholesteatoma within the attic has extended down into the middle ear. Note the attic crust and the white mass of cholesteatoma behind the posterior quadrant of the tympanic membrane. (Left ear)

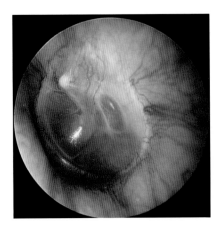

Figure 1.187
Glomus vagale

The large pink mass pressing against the inferior quadrant of this tympanic membrane arose from the vagus nerve. The portion of this glomus vagale that can be seen in the middle ear is just the 'tip of the iceberg'. (Left ear)

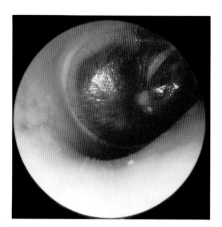

Figure 1.188
Glomus jugulare

The large bright-red mass filling the middle ear and pushing the tympanic membrane laterally is a huge glomus jugulare tumour. (Right ear)

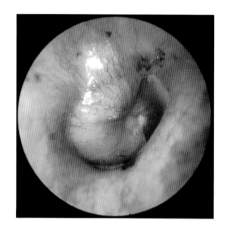

Figure 1.189
Primary adenoma of middle ear

The creamy-white mass filling the posterior four-fifths of this middle ear was a primary adenoma arising from the mucosal lining of the middle ear. (Right ear)

2 The nose

Introduction

The nasal symptoms of blockage, discharge, midfacial discomfort and abnormalities of the sense of smell are non–specific and do not correlate well with the different types of pathology that can present with these problems. Consequently, a complete and competent nasal examination is always required to establish the diagnosis.

External inspection of the nose may reveal deformity of the external nasal shape or suggest a significant deviation of the nasal septum. Facial scars from previous nasal and sinus surgery can often be missed, and careful inspection of the face and oral cavity is required. A rough guide to nasal airflow can be obtained from the nasal exhalation pattern on to a cold metal surface or a mirror. A strong light source (headlight or head mirror) is required to illuminate the interior of the nasal cavity.

The tip of the nose is everted and all areas of the nasal vestibule inspected. All areas of the nasal vestibule must be completely examined in order to avoid missing a small malignant tumour or papilloma 'hidden' within the vestibule. In children, eversion of the nasal tip may be all that is required to inspect adequately the anterior nasal cavity; in adults, opening the nasal vestibule and separating the nasal hairs with the insertion of a nasal speculum are required to inspect the nasal cavity. It is advisable to have a systematic technique of inspection (e.g. septum, nasal floor, inferior meatus, inferior turbinate, middle turbinate and roof of the nasal cavity) in order to identify all visible pathology. Application of a topical decongestant will reduce the size of the inferior turbinate and improve inspection of the nasal cavity.

The examination of the postnasal space with a mirror and headlight is often difficult in adults and generally both impossible and inadequate in young children. Fibreoptic nasal endoscopes, rigid-rod endoscopes and radiology are all important methods of assessing a patient's nasopharynx. A patient should be referred to a specialist with access to these forms of investigation when nasopharyngeal pathology is suspected.

An examination of the nose is never complete until the neck has been examined. Malignancy of the nose, paranasal sinuses and nasopharynx may have spread to the neck even when there are only minimal or even no nasal symptoms.

Nasal endoscopic examination with Hopkins rigid–rod endoscopes is now an integral and essential part of a complete nasal examination. The rigid endoscope enables the doctor to inspect the mucosal lining together with the clefts and recesses of the nasal cavity in great detail. In particular, the middle meatus and the region of the anterior ethmoid cells, a key area in the genesis of chronic paranasal sinus disease, can be inspected.

Functional Endoscopic Sinus Surgery (FESS) is based on concepts developed from original research into the anatomy and pathophysiology of the paranasal sinuses by Professor Walter Messerklinger. He established that the health of the frontal and maxillary sinuses was subordinate to the anterior ethmoids and, in particular, to the prechambers or channels of the frontal recess and the infundibulum. The major sinuses drain and ventilate through these prechambers of the frontal recess or infundibulum; he demonstrated that occlusion or narrowing of these channels was the prime cause of recurrent sinus infection.

Messerklinger noted in his patients that a limited endoscopic resection of the disease within the anterior ethmoid responsible for the obstruction of the ventilation and drainage pathways of these larger paranasal sinuses allowed re-establishment of ventilation and drainage through the natural pathways. The key principle of FESS is thus that a minimal localized resection of disease obstructing the ethmoidal prechambers allows restoration of normal mucociliary clearance and ventilation; this is followed by spontaneous resolution of the mucosal disease in the maxillary and frontal sinuses.

The role of Computed Tomography (CT) in the examination of the paranasal sinuses is important. An endoscopic examination demonstrates the 'surface' structures within the nasal cavity, whereas the CT scan demonstrates the delicate bony chambers of the ethmoidal labyrinth and helps to identify those anatomical variants that may compromise the ventilation and drainage of the paranasal sinuses and thus predispose the patient to recurrent episodes of sinusitis.

A systematic endoscopic examination of the lateral nasal wall in conjunction with a CT examination of the nose and paranasal sinuses will allow a precise localization of the underlying disease processes and thus aid the clinician in planning appropriate therapy.

External nose

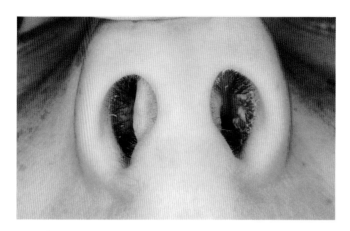

Figure 2.1
Caudal deviation of the nasal septum

The anterior end of the nasal septum in this patient has become displaced from its normal position in the columella. Deviations of the anterior or caudal margin of the nasal septum are called 'caudal deviations'.

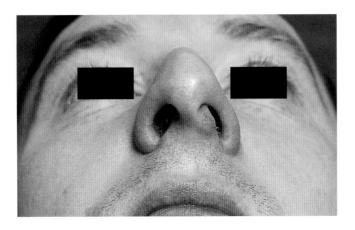

Figure 2.2
Septal dislocation

In this male patient there is a gross dislocation of the nasal septum into the left nasal vestibule; there is also an associated external twist to the lower half of the nose. Septal surgery to unblock the left nostril will require considerable technical expertise if it is to achieve a good functional and cosmetic result.

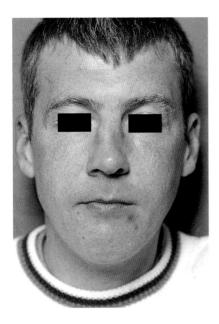

Figure 2.3
Nasal deformity

This male patient has been hit by a right fist; a characteristic left–sided nasal indentation and right–sided prominence has resulted. The nasal septum has a similar shape in response to the punch, with a caudal septal dislocation into the left nostril and a convex septal deformity in the right nostril. This patient requires a septorhinoplasty.

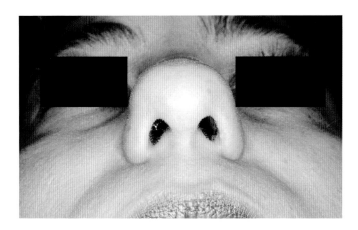

Figure 2.4
Alar collapse (during exhalation)

The alae nasi which make up the lateral walls of the nasal vestibule provide the rigid cartilaginous 'skeleton' that prevents the nasal vestibule from collapsing inwards during inspiration.

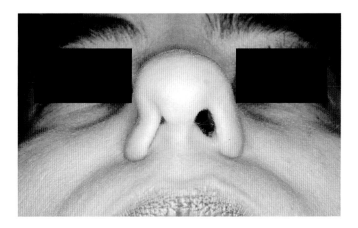

Figure 2.5
Alar collapse (during inspiration)

When the cartilaginous supporting framework within the ala nasi is weakened or deficient, the lateral wall of the nasal vestibule will be sucked inwards during nasal inspiration (alar collapse), as seen on this patient's right side.

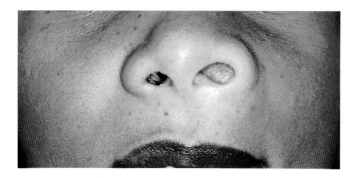

Figure 2.6
Nasoalveolar cyst (left nasal vestibule)

Nasoalveolar cysts form in the embryological line of fusion between the
lateral nasal process and the maxillary process. Clinically, a nasoalveolar
cyst presents as a smooth compressible swelling arising from the lateral
portion of the floor of the nasal vestibule. The large nasoalveolar cyst
seen in this patient obstructs the nasal vestibule and displaces the left
ala nasi and the nasolabial fold both laterally and anteriorly.

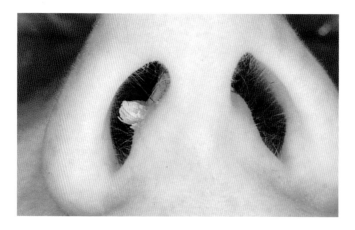

Figure 2.7
Benign squamous papilloma

Benign squamous papillomas are the most common benign tumours of
the nasal vestibule. They not infrequently seed on to adjacent areas of
the nasal septum, suggesting a viral aetiology.

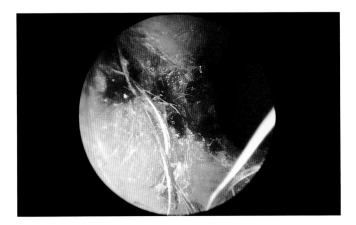

Figure 2.8
Nasal vestibulitis

'Nasal vestibulitis' is the term used to describe a chronic staphylococcal infection of the skin and hair follicles of the nasal vestibule. Nasal vestibulitis frequently develops as the result of local trauma to the skin of the nasal vestibule from repeated nasal picking. Yellowish crusts and scabs are usually seen starting at the base of the vestibular hairs (vibrissae) and extending on to the adjacent vestibular skin and nasal mucous membranes.

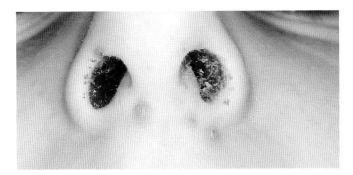

Figure 2.9
Impetigo

In impetigo contagiosa the causative organisms are usually either group A streptococci or *Staphylococcus aureus*. The thick yellowish crusts filling this right nasal vestibule and seeding on to the upper lip are characteristic of impetigo.

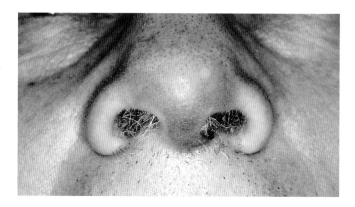

Figure 2.10
Cellulitis

The brawny-red painful swelling affecting the skin over the tip of this patient's nose indicates the presence of cellulitis.

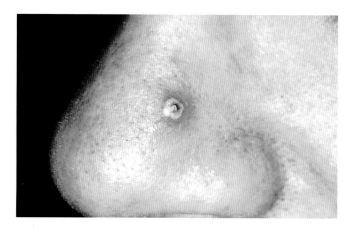

Figure 2.11
Furuncle

A furuncle or pimple is a small staphylococcal abscess that arises in the base of a hair follicle. All infections of the external nose must be treated aggressively to avoid the infection spreading to the cavernous sinus and producing a cavernous sinus thrombosis.

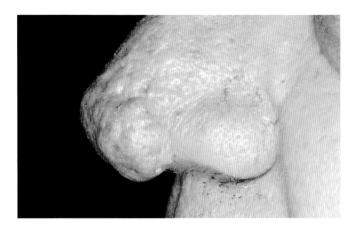

Figure 2.12
Rhinophyma

Rhinophyma is the result of a massive hyperplasia of the sebaceous glands of the nasal skin, which is often associated with acne rosacea. The result is a thickening and coarsening of the skin covering the lower cartilaginous portion of the nose. It is incorrect and unfair to associate rhinophyma with chronic alcoholism.

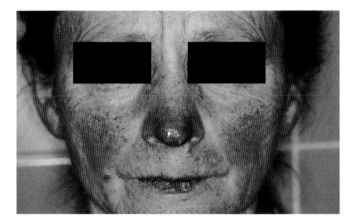

Figure 2.13
Sarcoidosis

The raised red infiltration of this nasal tip demonstrates the characteristic appearance of sarcoidosis.

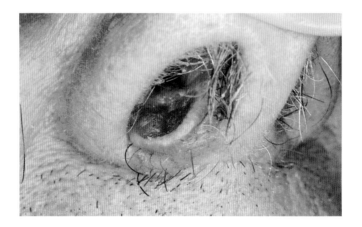

Figure 2.14
Squamous cell carcinoma of nasal vestibule

The ulcerated 'sore' in the floor of the right nasal vestibule was
initially treated as a case of nasal vestibulitis. A biopsy taken when
the lesion failed to heal revealed the presence of an ulcerated
squamous cell carcinoma.

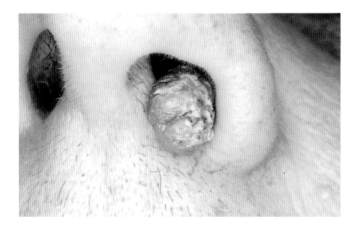

Figure 2.15
Carcinoma of nasal vestibule

A biopsy is indicated for any persistent or non-healing cutaneous
lesion. This relatively benign-appearing exophytic lesion arising from
the floor of the left nasal vestibule was a well-differentiated squamous
cell carcinoma.

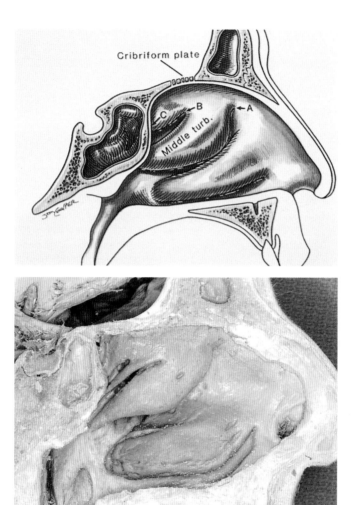

Figure 2.16
Lateral nasal wall

The nasal cavity's most important structures are situated on its lateral walls. Note the inferior turbinate, which occupies the inferior third of the lateral nasal wall. The middle turbinate and further superior subdivisions (the superior and the supreme turbinates) can be seen occupying the upper third of the lateral nasal wall. Note how the anterior end of the middle turbinate is located well behind and above the anterior end of the inferior turbinate. (Top) Diagram (courtesy of Dr M May) A, anterior insertion of middle turbinate; B, anterior insertion of superior turbinate; C, sphenoid sinus ostium; (bottom) gross specimen.

Nasal cavity

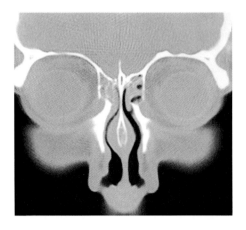

Figure 2.17
Nasal septal swell body

A discrete area of erectile tissue is present in the submucosa over the anterior cartilaginous nasal septum in most individuals. Vasodilatation of this 'septal swell body' can be a cause of significant nasal obstruction. A septal swell body may initially be confused with a deviation of the nasal septum; however, the septal body can easily be identified by palpation, since the erectile tissue can readily be compressed, unlike the cartilage of a septal deviation.

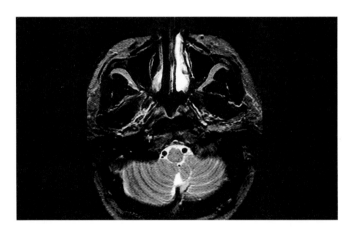

Figure 2.18
Normal nasal cycle

The state of vasodilatation (engorgement) and vasoconstriction of the erectile tissue of the inferior turbinate and of the nasal septal swell body normally alternates between the nasal cavities, i.e. as one side undergoes vasodilatation, the other becomes vasoconstricted. This is called the 'nasal cycle'. In this T2-weighted MRI scan, note the bright areas, which represent vasodilatation of the right inferior turbinate and nasal septum.

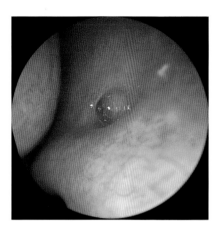

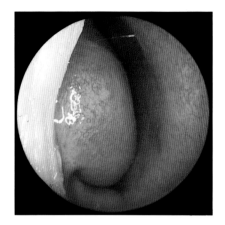

Figure 2.19
Jacobson's organ

A shallow circular pit or depression, which resembles a small ulcer or punched-out lesion, can sometimes be seen on the anterior cartilaginous nasal septum. This is 'Jacobson's organ', a vestigial olfactory organ that has no known function in humans. A Jacobson's organ should not be confused with a septal ulceration.

Figure 2.20
Normal inferior turbinate

The inferior turbinate is the lowest and most anterior of the three scroll-shaped nasal turbinates (inferior, middle and superior) located on the lateral walls of the nasal cavities. Its anterior border is the first intranasal structure encountered during a rhinoscopic examination. The submucosal layer of the inferior turbinate contains erectile tissue. The status of the nasal mucosa can be inferred from its colour: normal nasal mucous membranes have a healthy pink colour and appear slightly moist. (Left nostril)

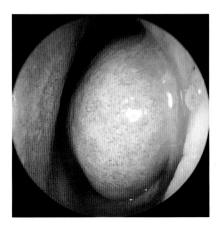

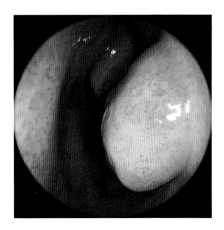

Figure 2.21
Swollen (vasodilated) inferior
turbinate

When the venous sinusoids within
the inferior turbinate are dilated, the
inferior turbinate may swell to such
an extent that it compromises nasal
respiration. (Left nostril)

Figure 2.22
Vasoconstricted inferior turbinate

A proper examination of the interior
of the nose cannot generally be
performed until the inferior
turbinates have been vasoconstricted
to allow access into the nasal cavity.
Vasoconstriction can readily be
achieved by the use of a topical
decongestant nasal drop or spray
such as 0.1% xylometazoline
hydrochloride nasal solution USP.
This is the same inferior turbinate
seen in Figure 2.21 approximately 10
minutes later. Note that the front
face of the middle turbinate can now
be seen posterosuperiorly. (Left
nostril)

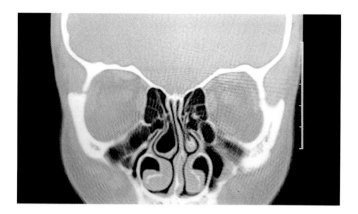

Figure 2.23
Normal vasodilatation of inferior turbinates

The erectile tissue within the nasal cavity, which is located primarily in the inferior turbinates, is usually in a state of partial vasodilatation. Note the size of the normal inferior turbinates on this coronal CT scan. The right turbinate is grossly enlarged owing to the presence of an abnormal air cell (a concha bullosa), which compromises the left middle meatus.

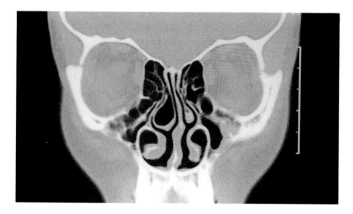

Figure 2.24
Vasoconstriction of inferior turbinates

This is the same patient as shown in Figure 2.23 approximately 10 minutes later. Note the change in size in the inferior turbinates following the application of a topical vasoconstrictor. A large concha bullosa of the right middle turbinate and bilateral Haller's cells are also present.

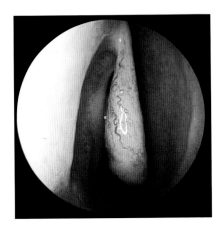

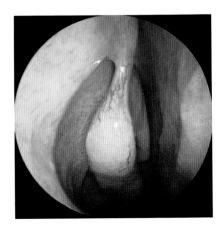

Figure 2.25
Normal right middle turbinate

The area lateral to the middle turbinate
is called the 'middle meatus'. Note the
insertion of the middle turbinate
(the neck of the middle turbinate) into
the lateral nasal wall. A normal middle
turbinate curves away from the lateral
nasal wall. The raised portion of the
lateral nasal wall which curves
medially to join the neck of the middle
turbinate is the 'lacrimal ridge'.

Figure 2.26
Normal right uncinate process

The curved structure that arises from
the lateral nasal wall just posterior to
the lacrimal ridge and extends
posteromedially like a visor over the
anterior aspect of the ethmoidal bulla
is the 'uncinate process'. The
ethmoidal bulla can be seen just
medial to the posterior edge of the
uncinate process.

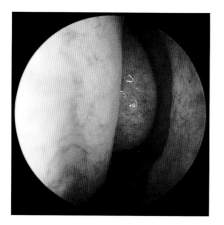

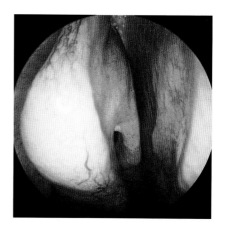

Figure 2.27
Ethmoidal bulla

The anterior ethmoidal bulla arises from the lamina papyracea just behind the uncinate process. The space between the posterior free margin of the uncinate process and the anterior surface of the ethmoidal bulla is the 'hiatus semilunaris'. In this patient the round structure seen behind the free margin of the uncinate process is a large ethmoidal bulla. (Right nostril)

Figure 2.28
Superior turbinate and superior meatus

The superior turbinate is a superior subdivision of the middle turbinate and not a separate anatomical structure. (Right nostril)

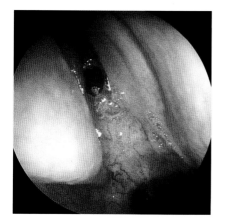

Figure 2.29
Sphenoid sinus ostium

The sphenoid sinus ostium is located in the posterosuperior portion of the nasal cavity just lateral to the insertion of the posterosuperior portion of the nasal septum into the anterior wall of the sphenoid. The right sphenoid sinus ostium can be seen between the nasal septum and the superior turbinate.

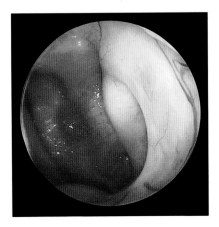

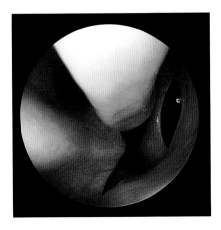

Figure 2.30
Eustachian tube

The torus tubarius (eustachian tube protrusion) is formed by the medial end of the eustachian tube, which projects into the lateral wall of the nasopharynx and consequently can only be seen by means of conventional posterior rhinoscopy (mirror examination of the nasopharynx) or, as in this case, by means of a nasal endoscope passed through the nasal cavity. The opening and closing of the torus tubarius can be observed as the patient swallows or performs a Valsalva manœuvre. (Left nostril)

Figure 2.31
Accessory maxillary sinus ostium

There are often defects in the medial wall of the maxillary sinus, part of the bony lateral wall of the nose. These defects in the bony skeleton are usually covered with a dense connective tissue that is a continuation of the periosteum. Accessory maxillary sinus ostia located in the anterior or posterior nasal fontanelles are not infrequently seen in the middle meatus. A small accessory ostium is present in the anterior nasal fontanelle on this left side. The uncinate process is bent medially.

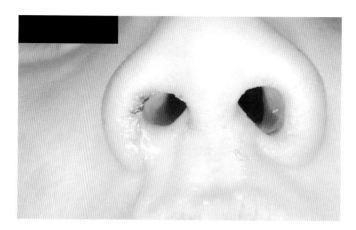

Figure 2.32
Foreign body

The presence of a persistent, unilateral, foul-smelling nasal discharge in a child often indicates the presence of a foreign body.

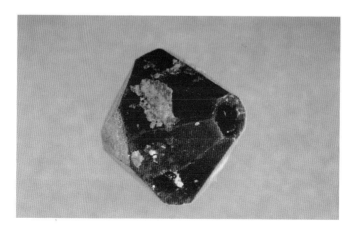

Figure 2.33
Foreign body

An inert foreign body such as this red plastic bead may remain inside the nasal cavity for a prolonged period of time without causing any symptoms.

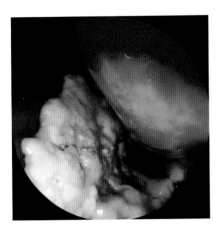

Figure 2.34
Rhinolith

If an inert foreign body remains
within the nasal cavity for many
years it may become surrounded by
a calcified coating. Such a 'nasal
stone' is termed a 'rhinolith'.
Rhinoliths may have a whitish-grey
colour, and are hard and gritty to
palpation; they are also radio-opaque
and can be clearly seen on an X–ray
or CT scan. (Left nostril)

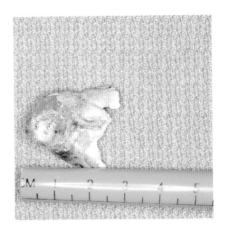

Figure 2.35
Rhinolith

Rhinoliths may 'grow' to a very large
size. This was the rhinolith removed
from the patient shown in Figure
2.34. Note the green plastic
tiddlywink, which was the nidus
around which the rhinolith formed.

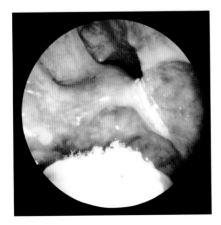

Figure 2.36
Maxillary sinus fungus ball

A fungus ball (non-invasive
Aspergillus fumigatus) was
encountered on the floor of this
sinus at maxillary sinoscopy. Clearly
visible are fungal spores mixed in the
mucopus, which is being transported
out of the sinus by the wide and
patent natural maxillary sinus
ostium.

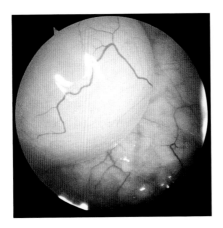

Figure 2.37
Maxillary sinus cyst

During sinoscopy a large cyst was seen arising from the roof of this maxillary sinus. The cyst was sitting on a dehiscent infraorbital nerve and was the cause of recurrent unilateral midfacial pain.

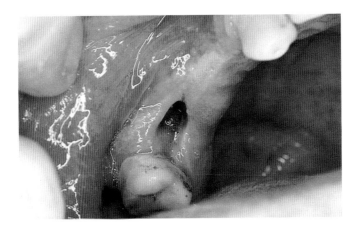

Figure 2.38
Oroantral fistula

A fistulous connection between the maxillary sinus and the oral cavity is called an 'oroantral fistula'. Oroantral fistulae are usually the result of the extraction of a tooth whose roots project into the maxillary sinus. This oroantral fistula (seen from below) was the cause of chronic suppurative maxillary sinusitis.

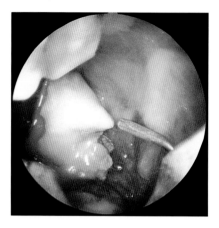

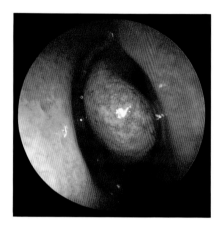

Figure 2.39
Oroantral fistula

Maxillary sinoscopy, on the left. An oroantral fistula developed following tooth extraction. The patient only visited the doctor weeks later, when an *Aspergillus mycosis* infection had developed in the sinus. The trocar sheath is visible at 7 and 5 o'clock; a probe is inserted through the fistula transorally. Note the pus-covered fungal concretions.

Figure 2.40
Acute viral rhinitis (URI)

During the prodromal phase of an acute upper respiratory infection (URI or coryza) the mucous membranes lining the nasal cavity are reddened, the nose is often abnormally patent, and the mucus is frequently scant and stringy in appearance. At this stage the patient usually complains of an itching or burning inside the nose. Shortly after, the mucosa becomes engorged and there is an outpouring of clear watery mucus.

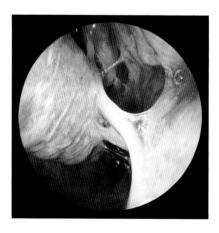

Figure 2.41
Acute viral rhinitis (URI)

If a bacterial superinfection develops, the mucus increases in amount and becomes coloured. As the acute phase resolves, the mucosa gradually returns to normal, although for a time there is still an overproduction of mucus, which at this stage is often abnormally viscid.

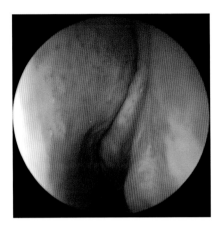

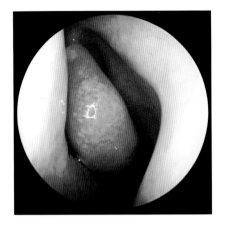

Figure 2.42
Rhinitis medicamentosa

The chronic use of topical nasal decongestants produces a state of chronic rhinitis, which is known as 'rhinitis medicamentosa'. Topical vasoconstrictors cause such severe constriction of the blood vessels of the nasal mucosa that ischaemic mucosal damage develops. Consequently, when the vasoconstrictor's effect wears off, the nasal mucosa 'rebounds', becoming reddened and oedematous. The patient then experiences increased nasal obstruction and reapplies the decongestant, thereby establishing a vicious cycle. On examination, the nasal mucous membranes are usually fiery-red and swollen. The history of topical decongestant abuse is usually freely given.

Figure 2.43
Vasomotor rhinitis

Vasomotor rhinitis is a common cause of chronic nasal congestion and rhinorrhoea, which is currently believed to be caused by an imbalance in the autonomic nerve supply to the nasal mucous membranes. Vasomotor rhinitis is characterized by chronic nasal congestion with engorgement of the inferior turbinates and by a troublesome profuse, clear and watery rhinorrhoea.

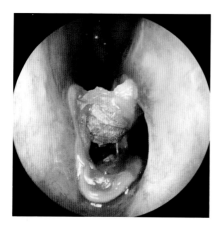

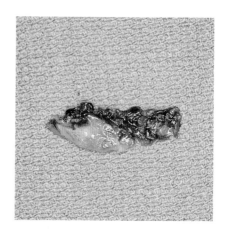

Figure 2.44
Atrophic rhinitis (ozena)

Atrophic rhinitis is an idiopathic,
chronic degenerative disorder that
affects both the nasal mucous
membranes and the turbinates. The
turbinates atrophy and the nasal
cavities consequently become
abnormally patent. Atrophic rhinitis
is characterized by the accumulation
of large greenish-yellow crusts and
severe fetor. Fortunately most of
these patients are anosmic. This
patient has iatrogenic atrophic
rhinitis, which developed following
excessive electrocautery to the left
inferior turbinate.

Figure 2.45
Atrophic rhinitis (ozena)

This large yellowish-green crust was
removed from the nasal cavity of the
patient in Figure 2.44. These foul-
smelling crusts result from the
associated acquired atrophy of the
cilia, which prevents the mucous
blanket from being carried normally
into the nasopharynx. The stagnant
infected mucus gradually dries into
the crust.

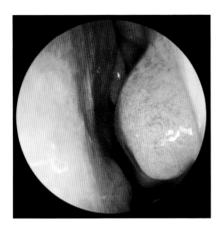

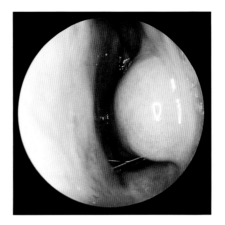

Figure 2.46
Allergic rhinitis

Because one of the main functions of the nose is the trapping and removal of particulate matter, it is not surprising that many individuals develop allergies to a variety of inspired substances. The allergic response within the nose results in a triad of symptoms: paroxysmal sneezing, nasal obstruction and a watery rhinorrhoea. This swollen bluish left inferior turbinate is pathognomonic for allergic rhinitis.

Figure 2.47
Allergic discolouration of nasal mucous membranes

The nasal mucous membranes in patients with allergic rhinitis often have a pale-blue, purple or even whitish coloration as seen in this swollen left inferior turbinate. Note the clear thin watery discharge.

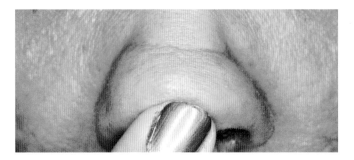

Figure 2.48
Allergic crease

The tendency of some allergic individuals to rub their itchy nose
repeatedly during childhood may produce a permanent horizontal skin
crease above the tip of the nose. This has been called the 'allergic crease'.

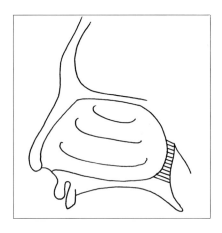

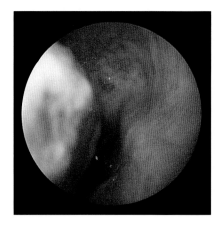

Figure 2.49
Choanal atresia

Choanal atresia is caused by a bony
or membranous congenital occlusion
of the posterior nasal opening—the
choana. Bilateral choanal atresia is a
severe and potentially life-threatening
emergency in the newborn, as the
newborn infant is obligated to be a
nasal breather and cannot breathe
with the mouth closed.

Figure 2.50
Choanal atresia

The blind pit of this women's right
posterior nasal cavity is shown. The
posterior end of the inferior turbinate
can be seen; note how the septum
curves laterally into the atresia. This
blockage was a bony (as opposed to
a membranous) atresia.

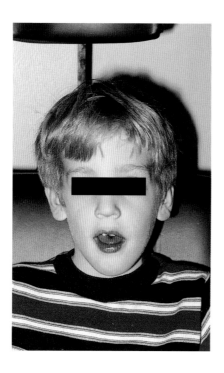

Figure 2.51
Adenoid facies

Hypertrophy of the nasopharyngeal pad of lymphoid tissue (the adenoids) is the most common cause of nasal obstruction in children. The most common presenting symptoms are chronic mouth breathing and snoring. The most dangerous symptom is sleep apnoea. Persistent mouth breathing due to nasal obstruction in childhood may result in the 'long face syndrome' (previously called 'adenoid facies').

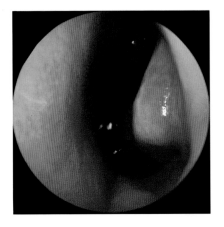

Figure 2.52
Anterior nasal mucosal changes:
nasopharyngeal obstruction from
enlarged adenoids

When the airflow through the nasal cavity ceases as a result of enlarged adenoids, a characteristic secondary change in the mucosa of the anterior nasal cavity may be observed. This change consists of a state of vasoconstriction and purple discolouration of the mucosa of the anterior portion of the inferior turbinates. These changes result in a wider than normal anterior air space and pale-purple small inferior turbinates. Such changes should not be misinterpreted as an allergic rhinitis.

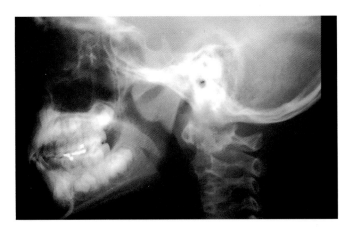

Figure 2.53
Adenoid hypertrophy (lateral radiograph)

Enlarged adenoids are not easily identified on physical examination. A lateral radiograph of the nasopharynx provides a simple and cost-effective method for assessing the size of the adenoids and the amount of postnasal air space remaining.

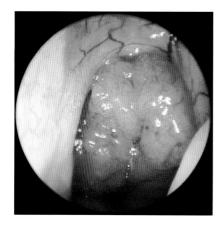

Figure 2.54
Adenoid hypertrophy (endoscopic view)

Enlarged adenoids extending anteriorly into and obstructing the left posterior choana are clearly seen on this endoscopic photograph of a 32-year-old man. While the adenoid tonsil usually undergoes spontaneous involution around puberty, the hypertrophy may persist into adult life. Adenoid hypertrophy in adults may be associated with HIV positivity.

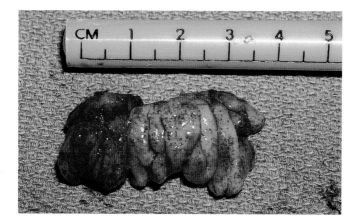

Figure 2.55
Adenoids (surgical specimen)

When obstruction of the nasopharynx causes total nasal obstruction, snoring, recurrent otitis media, secondary dental problems or sleep apnoea, then adenoidectomy is indicated. This huge adenoid tonsil was removed from the nasopharynx of a 6-year-old child.

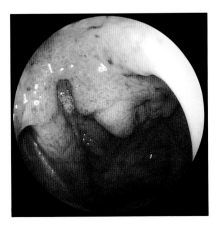

**Figure 2.56
Carcinoma of the
nasopharynx**

This 48-year-old man
presented with a history of
blood-tinged nasal mucus.
The area of 'adenoid tissue'
in the vault of the left
nasopharynx was proven to
be a carcinoma of the
nasopharynx by biopsy.

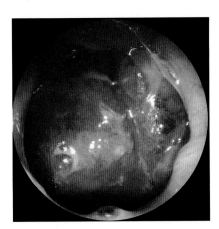

**Figure 2.57
Carcinoma of the
nasopharynx**

Transnasal view on to the
choana on the left side,
displaying a large
nasopharyngeal carcinoma.

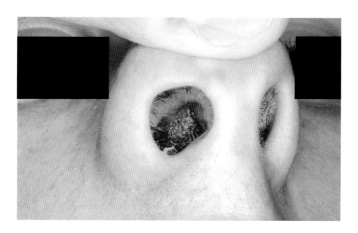

Figure 2.58
Nasal septal haematoma

Subperichondrial bleeding following trauma to the nose may produce a
collection of blood between the perichondrium and the underlying
cartilage of the nasal septum. The nose is characteristically blocked
and tender to palpation, especially when the nasal tip is elevated.
Prompt surgical drainage is required, because if the haematoma
persists or becomes infected, the cartilage will become necrotic and
the support provided by the anterior septal cartilage of the nose will
be lost, resulting in a 'saddle-nose' deformity.

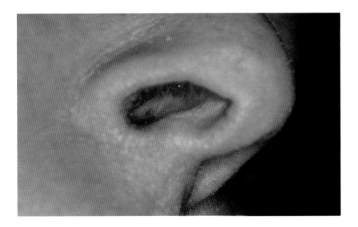

Figure 2.59
Cotton–tip abuse

This female patient had an irritation in her nasal vestibule which she
rubbed regularly with a cotton–tipped applicator. She has completely
abraded the mucosa over the nasal septum, and the underlying septal
cartilage is now exposed. Confiscation of cotton–tipped applicators and
the use of bland nasal ointment resolved the problem.

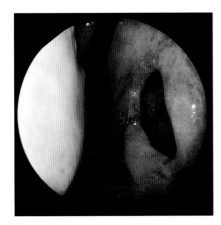

Figure 2.60
Nasal septal perforation

Perforations of the nasal septum may
occur from a variety of causes. The
most common cause is previous
septal surgery. Other causes include
nose picking, repeated cauterization
of the nasal septum for epistaxis,
exposure to industrial chemicals
such as chromium, repeated cocaine
abuse, nasal granulomas, and
chronic infections such as syphilis or
tuberculosis. Smaller septal
perforations are usually
asymptomatic, although they may
produce a whistling noise during
nasal respiration.

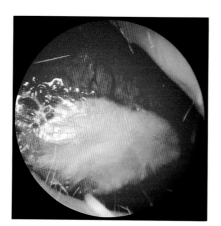

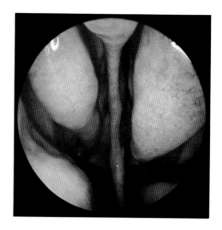

Figure 2.61
Hyperkeratosis of nasal septum

Chronic local trauma to the anterior
nasal septum from nose picking has
caused the mucosa of the anterior
nasal septum to undergo squamous
metaplasia producing a thickened
white hyperkeratotic area.

Figure 2.62
Large nasal septal perforation

Large septal perforations often
produce a sensation of nasal
stuffiness which is probably due to
airflow disturbance. The drying effect
of the inspired air on the posterior
margin of the perforation frequently
causes crust formation, and epistaxis
as the crusts separate. The mucosa of
the margins of the perforation
frequently undergo squamous
metaplasia and thus appear clinically
to be hyperkeratotic. This patient has
a huge nasal septal perforation
involving most of the nasal septum.
Both sides of the nose can be seen on
either side of the posterior remnant of
the nasal septum. The spontaneous
development of a nasal septal
perforation should always raise the
possibility of one of the two potentially
fatal non-healing granulomas of
unknown origin that may occur in the
nasal cavity: Wegener's
granulomatosis and midline malignant
non-healing granuloma.

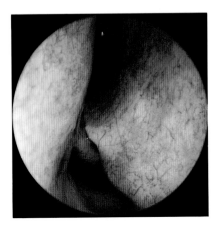

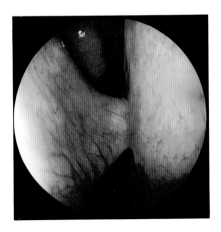

Figure 2.63
Severely deviated nasal septum

While the ideal nasal septum is located in the midline of the nasal cavity, most normal nasal septa deviate to a slight extent from the midline. Such minimal deviations do not interfere with airflow through the nose and should not be considered abnormal. Nasal septal deviations that are severe enough to affect nasal airflow are relatively common and usually involve the anterior half of the nasal septum. This patient's quadrilateral cartilage has deviated into the right nasal fossa to such an extent that nasal respiration has become severely limited. Any additional mucosal swelling (e.g. from allergic rhinitis or from an upper respiratory infection) will totally block the left nasal cavity.

Figure 2.64
Nasal septal spur

In this patient, probably as the result of a local growth disorder, the vomer has developed a spur, which presses into the left inferior turbinate and which was responsible for recurrent unilateral headaches.

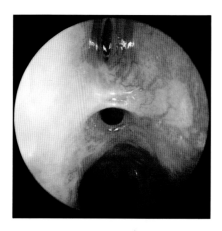

Figure 2.65
Synechiae

Synechiae are red or pale-pink
fibrous adhesions that usually run
across the nasal cavity between the
nasal septum and the inferior
turbinate. Synechiae develop
following an injury that creates
opposing raw surfaces on the lateral
nasal wall and the nasal septum.
The tiny synechia running between
this left middle turbinate and the
lacrimal ridge is of no clinical
significance. While most synechiae
are small and asymptomatic, on
some occasions synechiae may be
large enough to interfere with nasal
respiration. Note the extensive
synechiae between the septum and
the right lateral nasal wall that
developed after endonasal surgery.

Lateral nasal wall

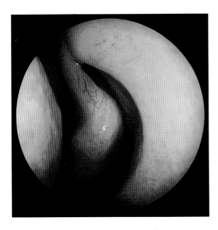 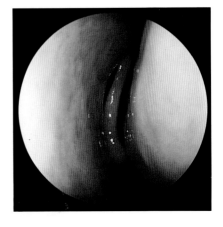

Figure 2.66
Paradoxically curved middle
turbinate

A normal middle turbinate curves
away from the lateral nasal wall, i.e.
the concavity of the middle turbinate
is directed laterally. This results in a
wide middle meatus. The concavity of
a paradoxically bent middle turbinate
is directed medially, with the
convexity of the middle turbinate
curving into the lateral nasal wall,
thereby narrowing the middle
meatus.

Figure 2.67
Lateralized middle turbinate

The middle turbinate may lateralize
or collapse laterally. In this case, an
atrophic right middle turbinate
appears to have been 'pushed'
laterally by a deviated nasal septum.
The middle turbinate has lateralized
to such an extent that the entrance
to the middle meatus is closed off.

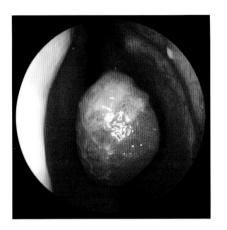

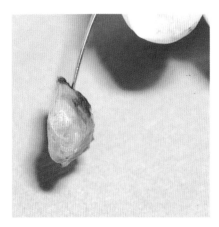

Figure 2.68
Anterior extending middle turbinate

The anterior face of the middle turbinate usually extends about 1 cm or less anterior to the point at which the turbinate inserts into the lateral nasal wall. In this patient, the head of the left middle turbinate extends anteriorly almost into the nasal vestibule.

Figure 2.69
Anterior extending middle turbinate

The anterior end of the left middle turbinate shown in Figure 2.68 was resected because it was causing significant obstruction to nasal respiration. The anterior face of the turbinate is seen on the left. The probe points to the level at which the turbinate inserted into the lateral nasal wall.

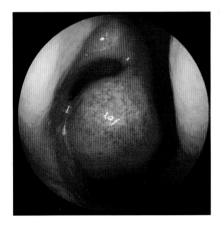

Figure 2.70
Concha bullosa

The normal middle turbinate consists of solid bone. When the bone of a middle turbinate contains an air cell it is called a 'concha bullosa'. The large air cell within this right middle turbinate has expanded the turbinate to such an extent that its lateral side has come into contact with the lateral nasal wall.

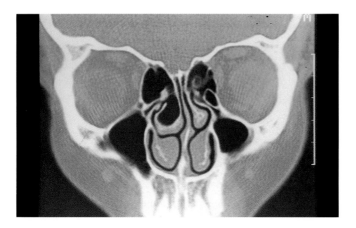

Figure 2.71
Concha bullosa

The large air cell within the right middle turbinate of the patient
shown in Figure 2.70 is clearly seen on the CT scan.

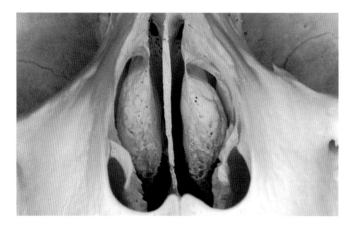

Figure 2.72
Concha bullosa

This specimen has bilateral large concha bullosa. Note the balloon-like
shape of both middle turbinates.

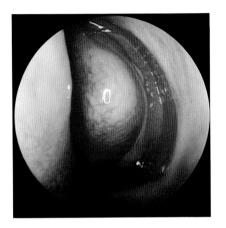

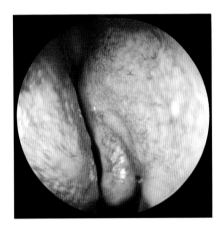

Figure 2.73
Concha bullosa

The air cell in this left middle
turbinate has expanded to such an
extent that the lateral surface of the
middle turbinate is now in direct
contact with the lateral nasal wall.
The middle meatus is obliterated by
oedematous polypoid mucosa that
developed at the site of contact.

Figure 2.74
Agger nasi

A pneumatized agger nasi mound
appears as a distinct bulge anterior
to the insertion of the middle
turbinate into the lateral nasal wall.
An enlarged or diseased agger nasi
may compromise the frontal recess
and cause frontal sinus disease. This
enlarged left agger nasi cell was
responsible for recurrent episodes of
frontal sinusitis.

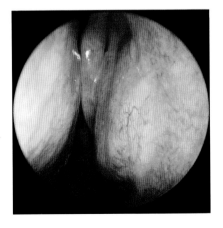

Figure 2.75
Enlarged and medially bent
uncinate process

In this patient with a left maxillary
sinus mucocele, the left uncinate
process is grossly enlarged and
rotated medially so that it lies at
right angles to the long axis of the
nasal cavity. The uncinate process is
so large that it obscures the anterior
surface of the ethmoidal bulla.

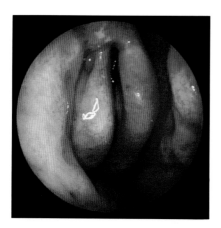

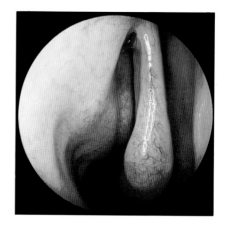

Figure 2.76
Anteriorly bent uncinate process

In some patients the uncinate
process is rotated almost 180°, so
that its posterior border faces
anteriorly. When the uncinate
process is also enlarged, as in this
patient, the middle turbinate appears
to be 'doubled'. The lateral 'extra
middle turbinate' is actually the
anteriorly rotated and enlarged
uncinate process, which protrudes
out of the middle nasal meatus.

Figure 2.77
Enlarged ethmoidal bulla

The ethmoidal bulla may be grossly
enlarged. In this patient the uncinate
process is both medially bent and
enlarged. The enlarged ethmoidal
bulla can be seen behind the medial
end of the uncinate process.

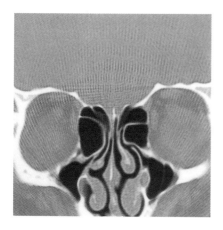

Figure 2.78
Enlarged ethmoidal bulla

Grossly enlarged ethmoidal bullae are
seen narrowing the ethmoidal
infundibulum bilaterally on this
coronal CT scan.

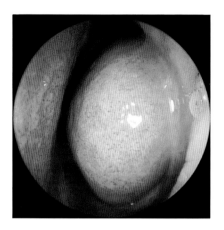
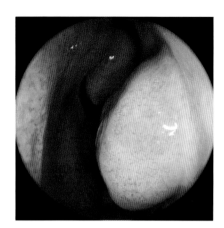

Figure 2.79
Enlarged inferior turbinate

'Enlargement' of the inferior turbinate is a common cause of nasal obstruction. In most cases, the apparent enlargement is primarily due to vasodilatation. Dilatation of the mucosa of the inferior turbinate may be the result of an acute or chronic rhinitis, or a reflex response to a focus of chronic infection or inflammation within the anterior ethmoid. In rare cases the underlying bone of the inferior turbinate is truly enlarged.

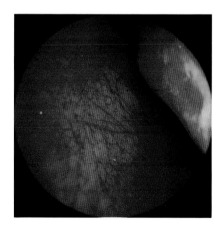

Figure 2.80
Epistaxis

Nosebleeds are extremely common and usually minor. Most nosebleeds originate from the anterior nasal septum in the highly vascular region of Little's area. Kiesselbach's plexus of vessels arises in Little's area of the nasal septum, from the termination of the major feeding systems: the anterior and posterior ethmoidal arteries, the septal branch of the superior labial artery and the sphenopalatine artery. Sometimes the vessels in Kiesselbach's plexus may become quite large and, by virtue of their superficial location, susceptible to damage from the most minimal trauma. The result is spontaneous recurrent episodes of epistaxis.

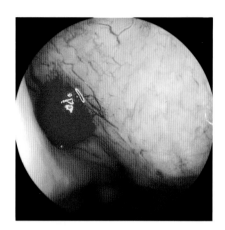

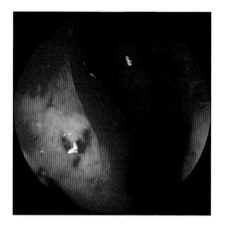

Figure 2.81
Epistaxis

The origin of the bleeding is not always obvious. Nasal endoscopes have proven invaluable for identification of the site of bleeding and for the application of site-specific cauterization. This small cherry-red haemangioma located on the anterior medial surface of this left ethmoidal bulla was the source of recurrent severe epistaxis. Once the haemangioma was identified, it was readily destroyed by suction electrocautery.

Figure 2.82
Rendu–Osler–Weber disease

Recurrent and troublesome epistaxis is a feature of congenital haemorrhagic telangiectasia (Rendu–Osler–Weber disease). Note the multiple telangiectatic spots on the anterior surface of this left inferior turbinate.

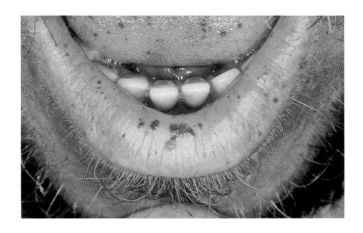

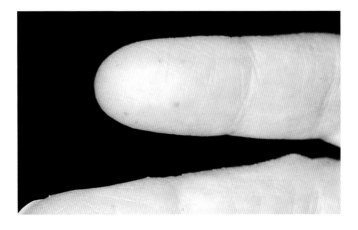

Figure 2.83
Rendu–Osler–Weber disease

Telltale telangiectatic spots may also be found on the surface of the lips, tongue and fingertips.

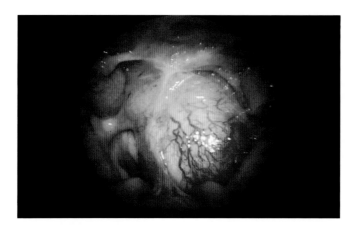

Figure 2.84
Juvenile angiofibroma

Recurrent episodes of epistaxis in adolescent males should alert the
examiner to the possibility of a juvenile angiofibroma. The left choana
of this 13-year-old boy is completely blocked by an angiofibroma. Note
how the nasal septum has been displaced to the right. (Courtesy of Dr
CT Buiter.)

Sinusitis

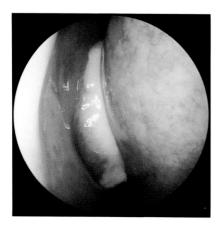

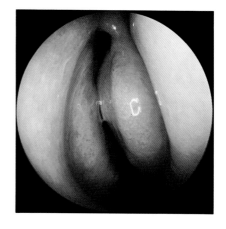

Figure 2.85
Acute maxillary sinusitis

Recurrent episodes of acute maxillary and frontal sinusitis are usually associated with significant anatomical abnormalities of the lateral nasal wall and osteomeatal complex. Note the creamy-white purulent discharge in the left middle meatus of this patient with acute bilateral maxillary sinusitis.

Figure 2.86
Acute maxillary sinusitis

The administration of a suitable broad-spectrum antibiotic is still the treatment of choice for acute, uncomplicated bacterial sinusitis. This is the same patient as shown in Figure 2.85, 5 weeks later. The predisposing anatomical abnormalities can now be clearly identified: a medially bent uncinate process and a concha bullosa. When medical therapy is unable to cure a sinus infection, then a functional endoscopic sinus surgical approach using the Messerklinger technique may be required.

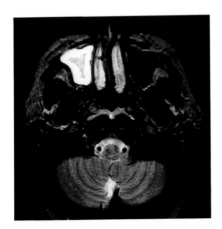

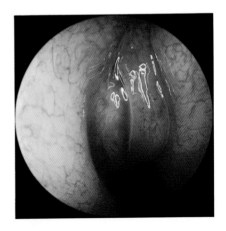

Figure 2.87
Acute maxillary sinusitis

The pathology with the maxillary
sinus during an acute sinusitis is
well demonstrated on this T2-
weighted MRI scan. Note the massive
oedema of the mucosal lining (the
brightest area) and the collection of
purulent material within the sinus
(less brightly illuminated).

Figure 2.88
AIDS-associated chronic sinusitis

Acquired immune deficiency
syndrome (AIDS) is associated with
an increased incidence of unusual
and potentially serious opportunistic
infections. This patient with AIDS
suffered from chronic pansinusitis.
Note the oedematous mucosa
herniating anteriorly from the right
hiatus semilunaris.

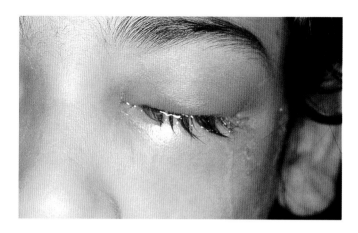

Figure 2.89
Orbital abscess

This young female patient presented with an acutely painful and swollen left eye. There was no visual difficulty. Treatment was with intravenous antibiotics.

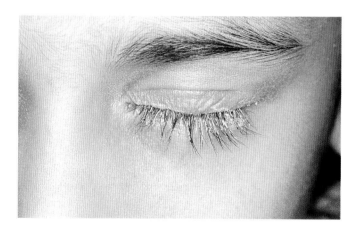

Figure 2.90
Orbital abscess

This photograph shows the result of 2 days of treatment by antibiotic for the resolution of the eye condition shown in Figure 2.89.

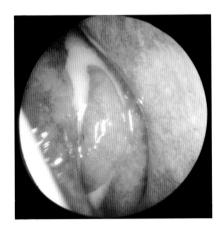

Figure 2.91
Orbital cellulitis

After cotton swabs soaked
with a decongestant
solution (adrenaline 1:1000)
were placed high up into
the middle meatus under
endoscopic control, pus
started to flow. Continuous
intravenous antibiotic
therapy was administered,
and complete resolution
occurred.

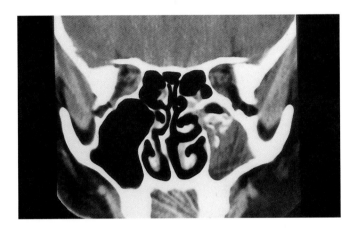

Figure 2.92
Fungal sinusitis

The presence of an area of increased radio-opacity on CT within the
paranasal sinuses indicated the presence of a fungal sinusitis (usually
due to *Aspergillus* species).

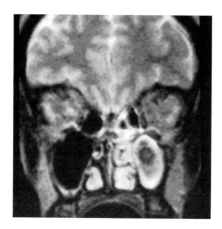

Figure 2.93
Fungal sinusitis

MRI scans can be used to confirm the presence of a fungal ball within a sinus cavity. The bright areas on this MRI scan of a left maxillary sinus represent inflamed and vascular mucosa. The central dark signal-void area represents the actual fungal ball.

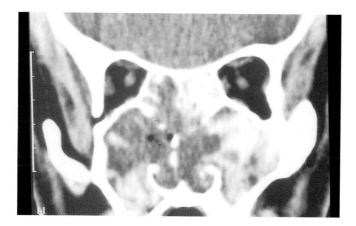

Figure 2.94
Allergic fungal sinusitis

While the aetiology of nasal polyps has yet to be fully understood, the role of allergy is undisputed. This patient with the ASA (acetylsalicylic acid) triad (asthma, nasal polyps and ASA sensitivity) has had four endonasal polypectomies in the past 14 months. After each polypectomy, the polyps recurred within 6 weeks. The reason for this rapid recurrence is suggested on this coronal CT scan. The streaky areas of increased radio-opacity within the maxillary sinuses and posterior ethmoid sinuses represent fungal elements.

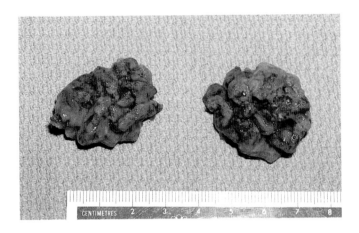

Figure 2.95
Allergic fungal sinusitis

This photograph shows the contents of the maxillary sinuses seen in
Figure 2.94. These khaki-coloured rubbery masses contained
numerous entrapped elements of the fungus *Aspergillus*. This material
is characteristic of patients with allergic fungal sinusitis. The allergic
reaction to the entrapped fungal elements was responsible for the
rapid recurrence of the nasal polyps. Not surprisingly, these nasal
polyps were highly steroid sensitive.

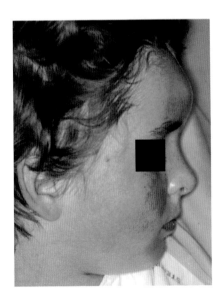

Figure 2.96
Frontal bone
osteomyelitis

Note the swollen forehead
in this 9-year-old girl with
frontoethmoidal sinusitis
that has extended into the
frontal bone causing
osteomyelitis.

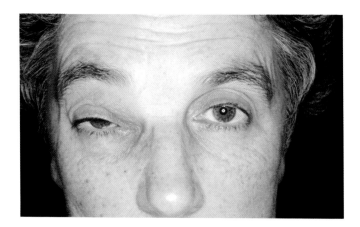

Figure 2.97
Frontal sinus mucocele with extension into orbit

The lateral and inferior displacement of this patient's globe was caused by a frontal sinus mucocele that had extended inferiorly into the anterior orbit and superiorly through the anterior skull base.

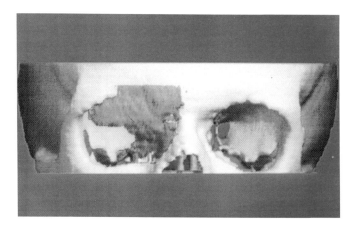

Figure 2.98
Frontal sinus mucocele with extension into the orbit

A three-dimensional reconstruction of the mucocele shown in Figure 2.97. The mucocele was decompressed by means of an endoscopic approach 7 years ago. To date, there has been no recurrence.

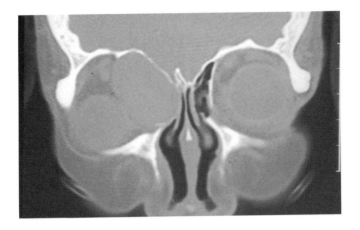

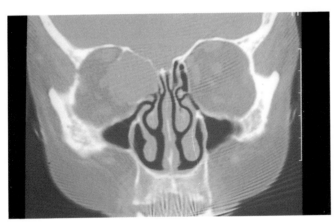

Figure 2.99
Anterior ethmoidal mucocele with extensive intraorbital extension

Note the large mucocele of the anterior ethmoid which has extended
extensively into the right orbit and caused severe displacement of the
globe.

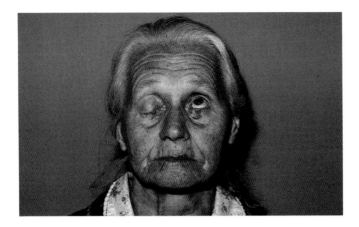

Figure 2.100
Posterior ethmoid and sphenoid mucocele

This 77-year-old patient developed complete ophthalmoplegia and blindness from a mucocele of the posterior ethmoid and sphenoid sinuses.

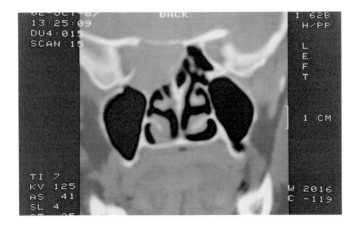

Figure 2.101
Posterior ethmoid and sphenoid sinus mucocele

The CT scan of the patient shown in Figure 2.100. Note the destruction of the lamina papyracea and the optic tubercle and the thinning of the bone at the sphenoidal/posterior ethmoidal roof. After endoscopic drainage, the ophthalmoplegia resolved; unfortunately, however, the vision did not return.

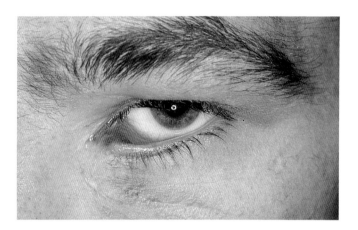

Figure 2.102
Lacrimal sac mucocele

This young man was involved in a road traffic accident which caused
an obstruction of his nasolacrimal sac. A lacrimal sac mucocele has
developed and can be seen expanding from an inferomedial direction
into the orbit. The scar from the initial injury can be seen below the
eye.

Polyps

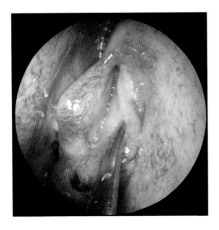

Figure 2.103
Nasal polyposis (polypoid rhinosinusitis)

A large polyp is seen blocking the entire anterior middle nasal meatus. When pushed medially, its origin from the contact area between the uncinate process and middle turbinate superiorly, with a broad root from the anterior face of the ethmoidal bulla, is apparent. The patient's symptoms were recurring maxillary sinus empyemas.

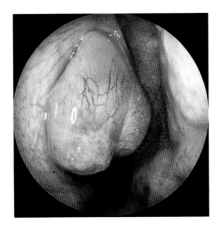

Figure 2.104
Nasal polyp

The large polyp extending anteriorly out of the right middle meatus has pushed the middle turbinate medially. The polyp has thinned the middle turbinate, apparently as a result of constant pressure against the septum. This polyp originated with a broad base from the free margin of a medially deflected uncinate process. No other pathology was encountered in the entire ethmoid during surgery.

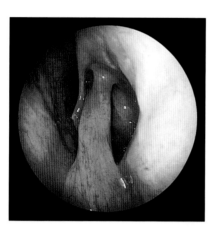

Figure 2.105
Nasal polyp

This large, oedematous, solitary nasal polyp arose by a small stalk from the superior portion of the uncinate process at its insertion into the middle turbinate.

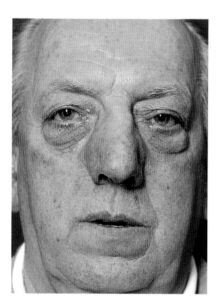

Figure 2.106
Nasal polyp

This male patient has had long–standing polyps which have caused a visible expansion of his entire nose.

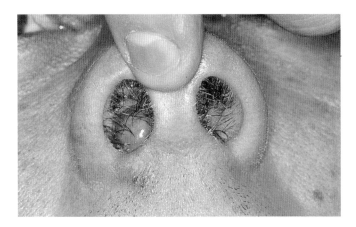

Figure 2.107
Nasal polyp

Eversion of the tip of this patient's nose shows the characteristic grey translucent appearance of a nasal polyp.

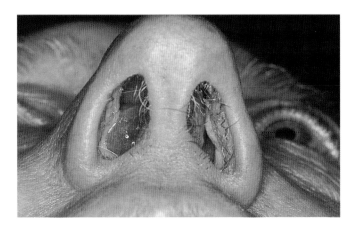

Figure 2.108
Nasal polyp

Eversion of the tip of the nose of the patient in Figure 2.106 also shows a nasal polyp but with a red appearance; the red appearance is due to metaplastic change at the tip of the polyp.

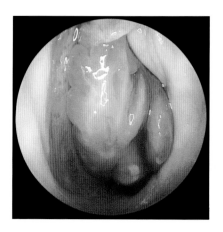

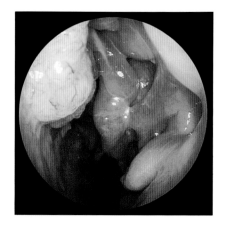

Figure 2.109
Steroid-sensitive nasal polyposis

The left nasal cavity of this patient
with massive nasal polyposis is
completely filled with oedematous
nasal polyps.

Figure 2.110
Steroid-sensitive nasal polyposis

Following a short course of high-dose
prednisone, the nasal polyps have
almost disappeared.

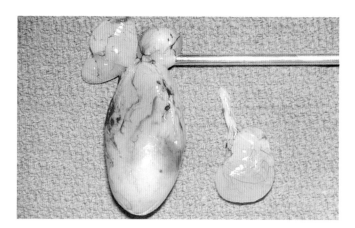

Figure 2.111
Nasal polyps

Nasal polyps can be removed endoscopically. Unfortunately, no matter
what technique is used for their removal, some nasal polyps have a
tendency to recur. The long-term use of a topical nasal spray seems to
slow their re-formation.

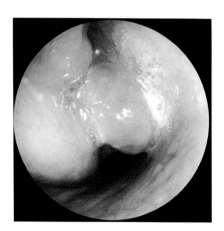

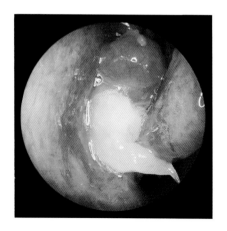

Figure 2.112
Nasal polyps and ASA triad

The typical appearance of the diffuse polypoid rhinosinopathy encountered in sinobronchial syndrome with the ASA triad.

Figure 2.113
Diffuse nasal polyposis and ASA triad

Patients with the ASA triad often have the most aggressive nasal polyps. Note the massive glue–like thick secretions below the polyps. This abnormally thick yellowish mucus is often associated with the ASA triad. The mucus may be so thick and rubbery in consistency that it may initially be confused with a nasal polyp.

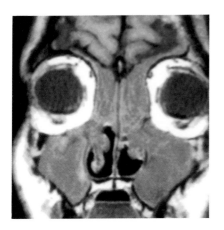

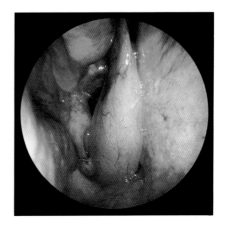

Figure 2.114
Aggressive diffuse nasal polyposis

Diffuse nasal polyposis represents a
diffuse mucosal disease (as opposed
to an area of diseased mucosa) and
as such it affects the mucosa lining
the entire nasal cavity and adjacent
paranasal sinuses. The diffuse nature
of this disease can be seen on this
T1-weighted MRI scan.

Figure 2.115
Choanal polyp

A large and often solitary nasal polyp
that blocks off the posterior nasal
choana is called a 'choanal polyp'. A
choanal polyp that arises from the
mucosa lining the maxillary sinus is
called an 'antrochoanal polyp'. Note
the large choanal polyp arising from
the medial surface of the left middle
turbinate.

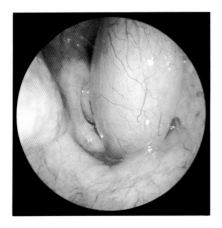

Figure 2.116
Choanal polyp

The inferior portion of the polyp
shown in Figure 2.115 extended
posteroinferiorly into the left nasal
choana.

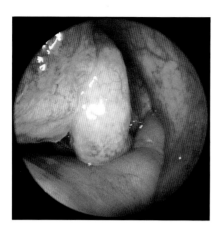

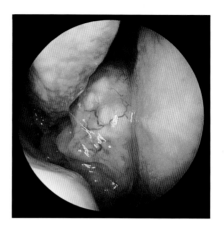

Figure 2.117
Choanal polyp

This patient had four or five discrete large nasal polyps in each nasal cavity. On the right side one of these large nasal polyps can be seen extending posteriorly along the floor of the nose and blocking the choana.

Figure 2.118
Inverting papilloma

This 45-year-old woman presented with a history of bilateral nasal obstruction. Endoscopic examination revealed an irregular polypoid mass arising from the left superior turbinate and extending anteriorly into the nasal cavity. On close inspection the surface of the polypoid mass has a knobby appearance suggestive of an inverting papilloma.

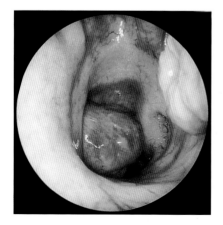

Figure 2.119
Inverting papilloma

The inverting papilloma shown in Figure 2.118 also extended through the nasopharynx to enter the right posterior choana. Inverting papillomas are 'benign' tumours that are locally aggressive and have a high incidence of recurrence.

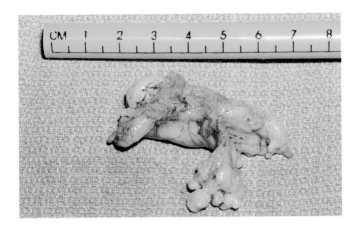

Figure 2.120
Inverting papilloma

The inverting papilloma shown in Figures 2.118 and 2.119 was
resected endoscopically. Note the knobby appearance characteristic of
an inverting papilloma.

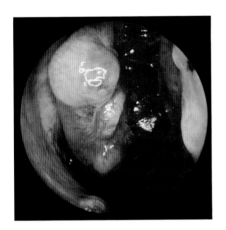

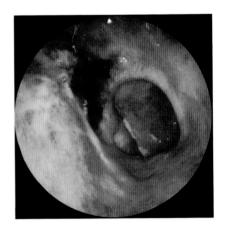

Figure 2.121
Olfactory aesthesioneuroblastoma

The salmon-coloured tumour seen
arising from the roof of the nasal
cavity and extending medial to this
right middle turbinate is an olfactory
aesthesioneuroblastoma.

Figure 2.122
Metastatic malignant melanoma

Malignant melanoma may metastasize
throughout the body. The
dark–brown spot arising from the
mucosa of the choana represents just
such an unfortunate event.

Postoperative appearances

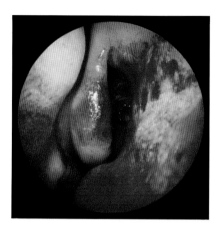

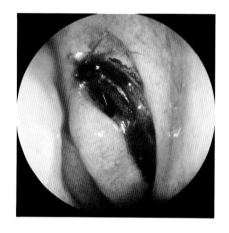

Figure 2.123
Postoperative appearance

The left middle meatus immediately after endoscopic ethmoid surgery.

Figure 2.124
Postoperative appearance

The entrance of a left middle meatus 6 days following functional endoscopic sinus surgery (FESS); there is normal healing. The secretions and crust are usually removed 1 week postoperatively.

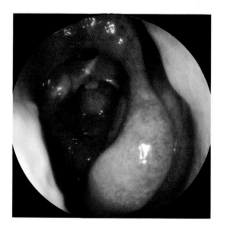

Figure 2.125
FESS

A right side showing the status 1 year after FESS. The frontal and maxillary sinuses now have free drainage and ventilation.

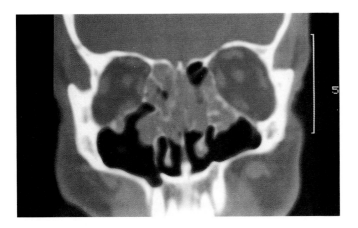

Figure 2.126
Inferior meatal antrostomy window with persistent anterior ethmoid disease

The CT scan of a patient who has undergone bilateral inferior meatal antrostomy (fenestration). The underlying pathology in the ethmoids, which was never treated, is clearly visible.

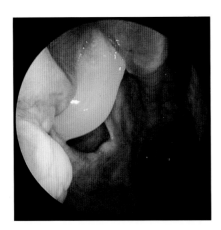

Figure 2.127
Inferior meatal antrostomy

A stream of white thick mucus can be seen recycling through this right maxillary sinus. The mucus leaves the sinus by its natural ostium, exits the hiatus semilunaris, and then slides inferiorly to re-enter the sinus by the inferior meatal window.

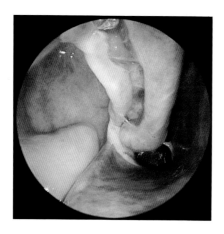

**Figure 2.128
Inferior meatal
antrostomy**

Despite the presence of a wide inferior meatal window, persistent disease within this maxillary sinus caused the accumulation of large amounts of thick green mucus within the sinus cavity, much to the patient's distress.

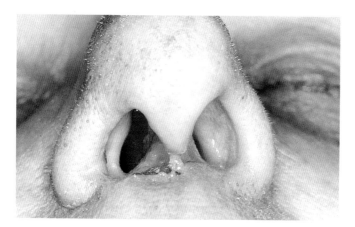

**Figure 2.129
Nasal septum radiotherapy damage**

This patient had a small squamous cell carcinoma of the anterior nasal vestibule that was treated by radical radiotherapy. The radiotherapy has caused the destruction and loss of the anterior nasal septum. Radiotherapy to a small head and neck tumour is sometimes said to produce a cosmetically superior result when compared to a surgical excision; as shown here, that statement is not always true.

3 The oral cavity

The practitioner should be able to perform a competent examination of the mouth.

- If the patient has dentures, these must be removed before the examination.
- A good source of illumination and a tongue depressor are required to allow a systematic exposure and inspection of all areas of the oral cavity.
- A gloved finger should palpate any suspicious area within the mouth. In particular, if the patient reports that there is 'something there', then the suspicious area in the mouth should be palpated even when no lesion can be seen.

Lips

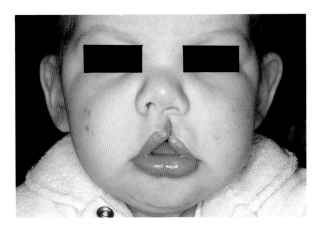

Figure 3.1
Cleft lip

A cleft lip is frequently associated with a cleft palate. The cleft in the lip is usually repaired at around the age of 3 months, whereas any associated cleft of the palate is repaired at a a later second operation. Despite meticulous surgical technique, there is always a degree of residual lip scarring. Associated deformities of the nasal tip and nasal septum may require surgery in later life, both to improve cosmesis and to relieve nasal congestion. Note the flattening of the left lower cartilage and the deviation of the nasal septum to the patient's left.

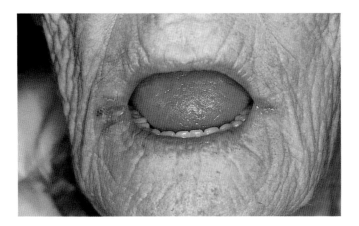

Figure 3.2
Angular cheilitis (angular stomatitis)

'Angular cheilitis' is the name given to the red fissures that develop at
the corner of the mouth. These localized areas of dermatitis arise as a
result of overclosure of the mouth or the ill–fit of dentures. Saliva
leaks out of the corner of the mouth, macerates the local skin and
promotes a localized monilial infection. Bland ointments, antifungal
medication, correction of dietary and haematological deficiencies and
the refit of dentures form the mainstay of treatment.

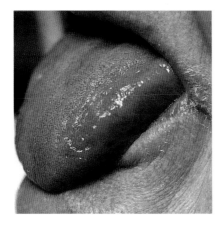

Figure 3.3
Angular cheilitis

The beefy red tongue of
atrophic glossitis is seen
in association with an
angular cheilitis due to
iron deficiency anaemia. In
this example the 'beefy'
appearance is located
predominantly on the
lateral border of the
tongue. Vitamin B
deficiencies and
megaloblastic anaemia are
often associated with
angular cheilitis.

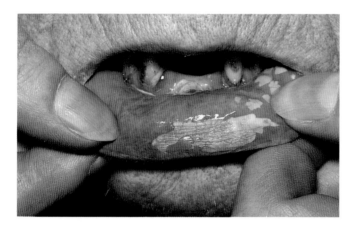

Figure 3.4
Hyperkeratosis of lip (leucoplakia)

'Leucoplakia' is a confusing but commonly used term to describe a
white patch of the oral cavity that cannot be wiped off and is not
susceptible to any other clinical diagnosis. Biopsy is always required
to reach a histological diagnosis. Leucoplakia on the vermilion surface
of the lip typically arises from excessive exposure to sunlight or from
the chronic thermal injury caused by the heat of a pipe stem. The
affected areas can be excised by a lip shave: the lip epithelium is
elevated from the vermilion–cutaneous border and the diseased
epithelium shaved from the lip prior to the advancement and suture of
the oral mucosa to the vermilion–cutaneous border. Regular
observation is required when the biopsy is negative for malignancy
and the lesion has not been excised.

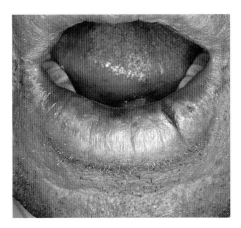

Figure 3.5
Lip fissure

This patient developed a split of the lower lip (fissure) as a result of exposure to a very dry environment; the lips are also dry and white. These changes can be prevented by the regular application of petroleum jelly.

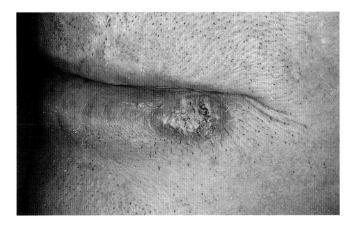

Figure 3.6
Squamous cell carcinoma of lip

Squamous cell carcinoma of the lip is characterized by a painless, infiltrative and hard sore (ulcer) occurring most typically on the lower lip. Predisposing factors are chronic irritation, solar radiation, leucoplakia and solar keratosis. Referral for biopsy is essential for any patient who has a persistent ulcer of the lip that has not healed within 1 month. Surgical excision consisting of a wide wedge–shaped resection with tumour–free margins is usually the treatment of choice.

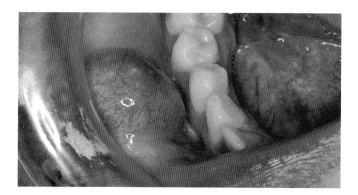

Figure 3.7
Mucocele of lip

The firm, indentable and somewhat translucent swelling of this lower
lip is a mucocele. A mucocele develops when the duct of one of the
mucous secreting glands within the lip becomes damaged by minor
trauma. The appropriate treatment is excision of the entire lesion
together with the remaining lobules of the associated gland.

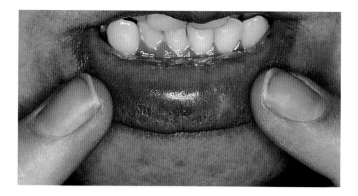

Figure 3.8
Melanonaevus

Pigmented lesions of the lip occur in hereditary haemorrhagic
telangiectasia, vascular malformations, Addison's disease and
Peutz–Jegher's syndrome. In this illustration the pigmented lesion of
the lower lip is a simple benign melanonaevus. Such a melanonaevus
is not uncommon.

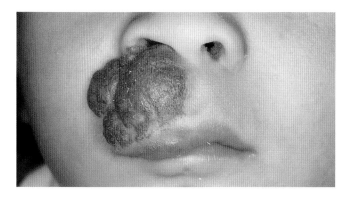

Figure 3.9
Haemangioma

A haemangioma is a congenital benign vascular tumour consisting of a mass of blood vessels. This child has a strawberry haemangioma of the upper lip. A strawberry haemangioma is raised above the surrounding tissue, blanches on pressure and is the most common type of haemangioma. Most strawberry haemangiomas are capillary in nature and tend to involute spontaneously by the fifth year of age.

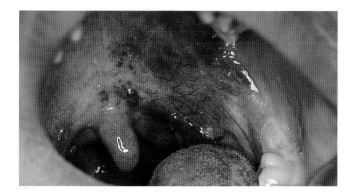

Figure 3.10
Vascular malformation of lip and palate

Vascular malformations of the lip and palate are rare. The malformation shown in this illustration extends from the lip posteriorly into the soft palate. Occasionally, severe bleeding may arise from such a malformation. Cryosurgery, laser therapy and ligation of feeding blood vessels may all have a role in the management of the patient with such a lesion.

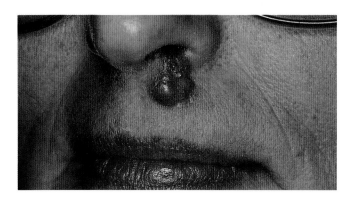

Figure 3.11
Herpes labialis (cold sore)

The small, initially painless cluster of clear vesicles on the lip of this woman is caused by the herpes simplex virus and is known as herpes labialis or 'cold sore'. Untreated, the vesicles rupture, crack and crust, producing considerable local discomfort. Treatment includes the use of alcohol–impregnated swabs to dry the lesions and the early application of acyclovir, an antiviral topical ointment.

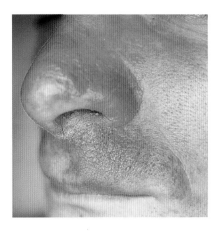

Figure 3.12
Crohn's disease of lip

Oral Crohn's disease and the related orofacial granulomatosis can produce swelling in the face, typically the lower lip. Obstruction of local lymph node drainage is considered the predisposing pathology. In this atypical example, the red and swollen discolouration of the upper lip shown was caused by Crohn's disease.

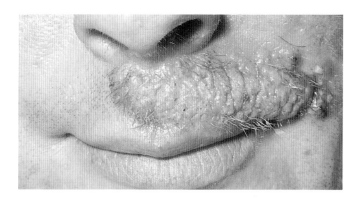

Figure 3.13
Ringworm of lip

A dermatophytic infection of the skin such as ringworm can affect the lip. The extensive swelling and induration of this upper lip is due to a tinea or ringworm infection.

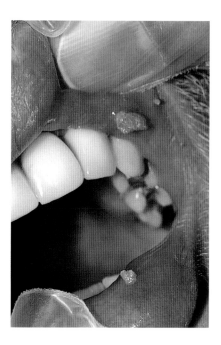

Figure 3.14
Papilloma of lip

A benign squamous cell papilloma of the lip often has a characteristic warty appearance and is probably of viral origin. The squamous papillomas of these lips were associated with genital warts; although most papillomas on the lips are not associated with genital warts, examination with a gloved finger is sensible.

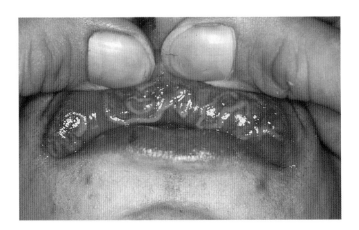

Figure 3.15
Syphilis (secondary mucous patches of lip)

'Snail track' ulcers or oral mucous patches are characteristic of secondary syphilis and are commonly seen on the hard palate. This patient is demonstrating his own 'snail tracks' of the upper lip (hence the lack of gloved fingers); such lesions are more commonly seen on the palate.

Teeth

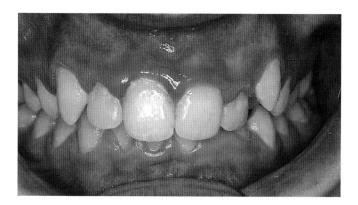

Figure 3.16
Gingivitis

Gingivitis or infection of the gums (gingivae) is common. In this
example, the gingival papillae have a slightly swollen, smooth, shiny,
red appearance. Most gingivitis is due to poor oral hygiene with an
accumulation of bacterial plaque on the teeth. Proper oral hygiene and
regular dental check–ups are required.

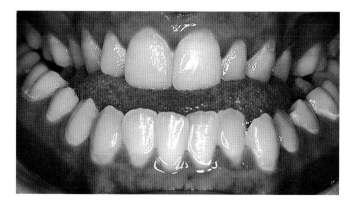

Figure 3.17
Gingivitis

The red, haemorrhagic areas seen in both gums are chronic gingivitis,
which resulted from poor oral hygiene. There is marked class III
malocclusion, which is caused by a discrepancy in the anteroposterior
position of the upper and the lower jaws.

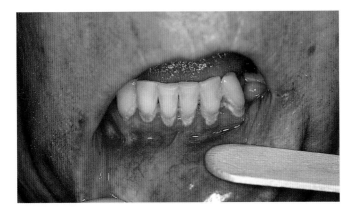

Figure 3.18
Dental caries

Dental caries is the gradual decay and disintegration of a tooth with
progressive decalcification of the enamel and dentine. The starting
point for caries is defects in the surface of the tooth. Decalcifying
acids are produced by the action of bacteria within plaque on trapped
carbohydrates. Moderate caries is visible around the roots of the teeth
in this illustration.

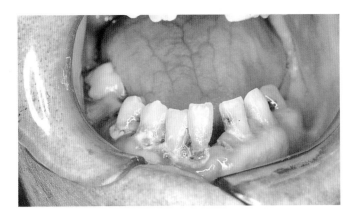

Figure 3.19
Dental calculus

The accumulation of scale or dental calculus around the roots of the
teeth is a characteristic feature of poor dental hygiene. Note the
associated gingivitis.

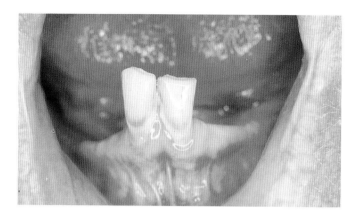

Figure 3.20
Mandibular resorption

The mandible and its teeth have a symbiotic relationship. Note the severe resorption of the mandible that has developed in those areas where there are no longer any teeth.

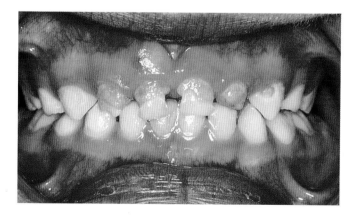

Figure 3.21
Childhood dental caries (bottle mouth)

Widespread decay (caries) of the deciduous dentition in this 5–year–old girl resulted from excessive and frequent ingestion of sugary drinks at night from a feeding bottle ('bottle mouth'). Dental extraction of the decayed teeth under general anaesthetic was required.

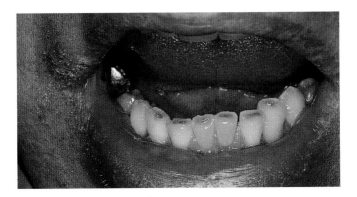

Figure 3.22
Dental abrasion

'Dental abrasion' is the term used to describe loss of teeth substance
as a result of extrinsic, usually chronic, minor trauma. This man
always gripped his pipe in the right-hand side of his mouth and this
has worn down the crowns of those teeth that held his pipe.

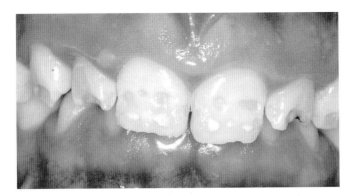

Figure 3.23
Dental hypoplasia

This 14-year-old girl suffered measles as an infant. The rubella
infection interfered with the formation of that portion of her
permanent teeth that was actively being developed at the time of the
illness. Consequently the earlier-forming upper central incisors are
affected halfway down the crown, whereas the later-forming lateral
incisors are affected at the tip. Veneers (porcelain facings) are required
to improve the unsightly appearance of these teeth.

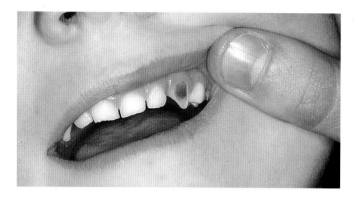

Figure 3.24
Discoloured teeth

Local trauma such as a fall on to or a blow to a tooth can result in devitalization and a consequent alteration in colour. Trauma to this child's left upper canine tooth has resulted in local discolouration.

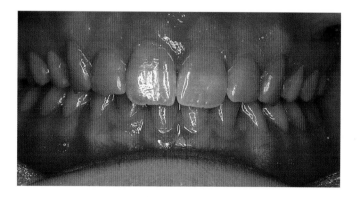

Figure 3.25
Tetracycline staining

This patient was prescribed systemic tetracycline during the period when her tooth buds were forming. This has resulted in discolouration of the permanent teeth. The tetracycline antibiotic group should be avoided in children under 10 years of age.

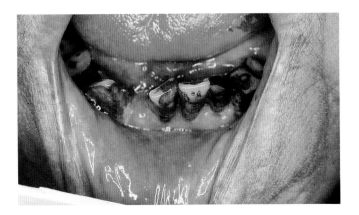

Figure 3.26
Betel nut stain

In some countries the chewing of a mixture composed of betel nuts, tobacco and slaked lime is a popular pastime. The black staining of the lower teeth in this photograph has arisen from that habit. Betel nuts are carcinogenic to the oral mucous membranes and predispose to leucoplakia and squamous cell carcinoma of the oral cavity.

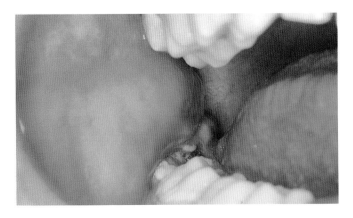

Figure 3.27
Pericoronitis: lower third molar

The thinning mucosal flap overlying an erupting third molar tooth has been traumatized recurrently by an upper molar tooth. This is termed 'pericoronitis'. Treatment may require removal of the upper tooth that is causing the trauma.

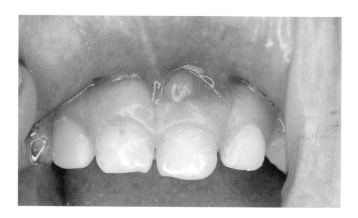

Figure 3.28
Dental abscess

Neglected dental caries can lead to infection in the pulp of a tooth with the subsequent death of the pulp of the tooth and local abscess formation at the tooth root. The patient usually presents with a swollen tender gum around the affected tooth and signs of systemic upset. The 'point' or site of eruption, however, depends on the local anatomy. In this example the swelling overlying the root of the upper incisor tooth is the presentation of a periapical abscess of that tooth.

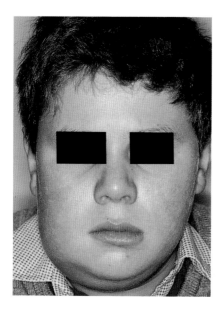

Figure 3.29
Dental abscess

In this illustration a molar tooth abscess has presented as facial swelling of the lower right–hand side of this young male patient's face. Such swelling is pathognomonic of a molar tooth abscess.

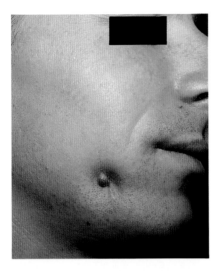

Figure 3.30
Facial sinus from dental abscess

When infection from a dental
abscess, such as that shown in
Figure 3.29, localizes either as a
result of antibiotic therapy or
spontaneously, an external sinus can
develop. Such a sinus, when
established, can be a source of
misdiagnosis. The nodule on the
cheek of this man could be mistaken
for a cutaneous tumour.

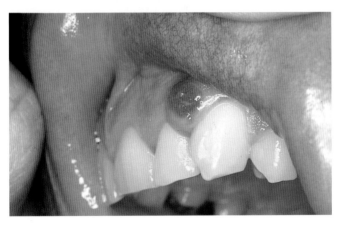

Figure 3.31
Epulis (pyogenic granuloma)

The gingival tissues are very susceptible to the development of
exuberant inflammatory overgrowths (epulides). These overgrowths
usually contain immature, vascular granulation tissue. The
classification of an epulis is determined by a combination of its
histological and aetiological factors. Pregnancy increases the
predisposition to form an epulis. In this illustration an infective
aetiology is proposed and the lesion is termed a 'pyogenic granuloma'.
The smooth pink swelling with the central area of protruding
granulation tissue is the pyogenic granuloma.

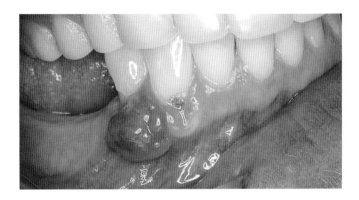

Figure 3.32
Epulis (peripheral giant cell granuloma)

The red-to-purplish swelling on the lower gingivae was diagnosed as a
peripheral giant cell granuloma by the demonstration of osteoclast-like
giant cells on histological examination. The exclusion of
hyperparathyroidism is required in this situation. Histological examination
is usually required to establish the diagnosis of most epulides.

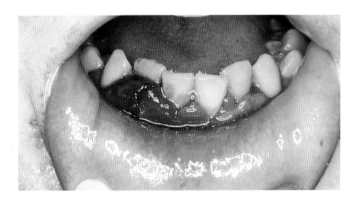

Figure 3.33
Gingival infiltration (leukaemia)

Enlargement and inflammation of the gingivae can occur during the
hormonal changes of puberty or pregnancy. Drugs such as phenytoin,
cyclosporin and nifedipine can all produce gingival hypertrophy.
Arguably the most important diagnosis to recognize, however, is that
which occurs with leukaemic infiltration of the gingivae. The bluish
haemorrhagic infiltration of these lower gingivae is due to an acute
myelomonocytic leukaemia.

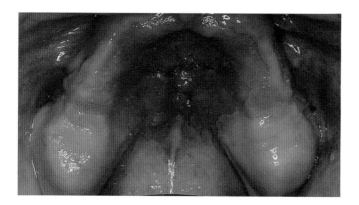

Figure 3.34
Denture granuloma

An ill-fitting denture can cause recurrent local trauma and irritation of
the mucosa of the mouth. This chronic irritation can incite a
connective tissue response resulting in a local overgrowth of tissue. In
this first example, there is a polypoid thickening of the upper gingival
soft tissue combined with an excess of tissue in the midline of the
palate. This patient also has very large maxillary tuberosities.

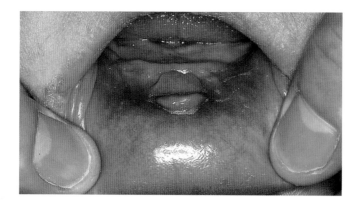

Figure 3.35
Denture granuloma

A loose–fitting lower denture has created a flange of organized
granulation tissue protruding from the middle of the base of the lower
lip/gingival margin. Removal of the granulation tissue combined with a
refit of the dentures is required.

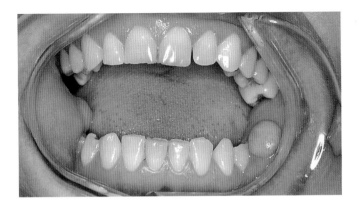

Figure 3.36
Fibroepithelial polyp

The smooth, pink, firm, sessile, benign polyp at each corner of this
patient's mouth (commissure) are fibroepithelial polyps. They have
arisen because of mild but chronic frictional trauma from the teeth.
Fibroepithelial polyps often develop a white surface.

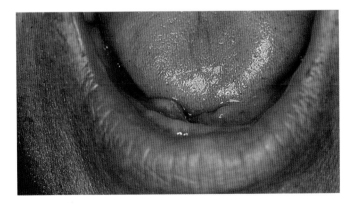

Figure 3.37
Torus mandibularis

A torus mandibularis is a smooth, hard, bony swelling that protrudes
characteristically from the lingual surface of the mandible in the
premolar region. A torus mandibularis composed of compact lamellar
bone is a benign lesion. The two smooth, bony protuberances arising
from the mandible and pointed to by the tip of the tongue are tori.
The edentulous lower mandible can also be seen.

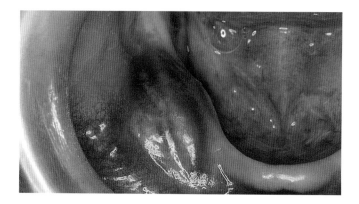

Figure 3.38
Odontogenic keratocyst

An odontogenic keratocyst is a keratin-containing cyst that most
commonly occurs at the angle of the mandible. This example shows a
characteristic smooth and slightly indentable swelling of the lower
mandible. Such cysts, when they occur in the maxilla, have a
tendency to rupture and discharge keratin.

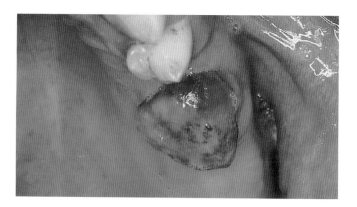

Figure 3.39
Antral mucosal prolapse through tooth socket

Sometimes after the extraction of an upper tooth, particularly a molar,
a fistula can arise between the mouth and the maxillary sinus. Antral
mucosa can then prolapse through the fistula producing a smooth,
pink, compressible swelling protruding from a tooth socket, as shown
in this illustration. Trimming of the antral mucosa and surgical
closure of the fistula are required.

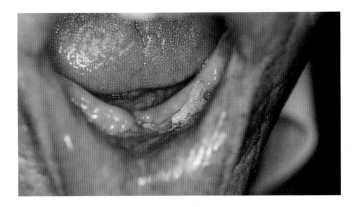

Figure 3.40
Exposed mandibular bone from radiotherapy necrosis

This patient received extensive radiotherapy to treat a squamous cell carcinoma of the left tonsil. The patient developed osteoradionecrosis of the mandible, which was subsequently revealed when the mucosa over the edentulous lower mandible broke down and a piece of necrotic bone (sequestrum) was exposed. Surgical excision of the sequestrum is appropriate, but if osteonecrosis of the mandible is widespread this can be an extremely difficult problem to resolve and spontaneous fracture of the mandible may occur.

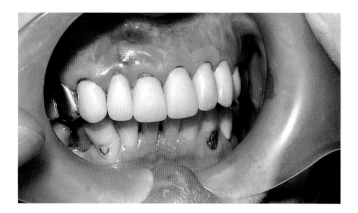

Figure 3.41
Amalgam tattoo

The blue discolouration of the gingiva arose from some recent dental work in which an adjacent tooth was filled with dental amalgam. Occasionally, isolated amalgam spots can be mistaken for an intradermal melanonaevus or even for a small melanoma. A dental radiograph will often demonstrate calcification in an amalgam tattoo and thus prevent an unnecessary surgical excision.

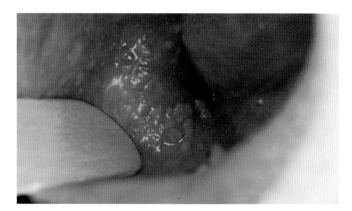

Figure 3.42
Fordyce spots

The yellow, slightly raised spots demonstrated on the inner mucosal surface of the cheek are prominent but normal sebaceous glands known as 'Fordyce spots'. This is a normal finding.

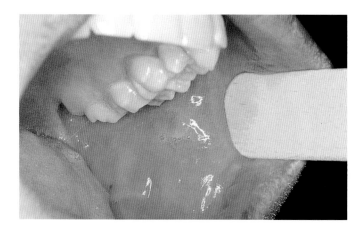

Figure 3.43
Parotid duct papilla

The parotid duct opens into the oral cavity through the buccal mucosa
approximately opposite the second upper molar. The raised area with
the central red section at the distal end of the wooden spatula is a
normal parotid duct papilla. Stroking this area with the tip of the
spatula often produces a flow of saliva.

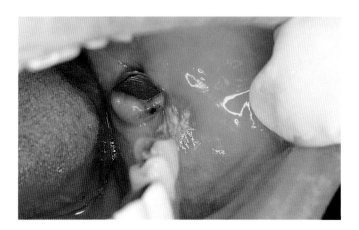

Figure 3.44
Leucoplakia

'Leucoplakia' is a descriptive term for a white patch on the oral
mucosa that cannot be wiped off and is not explicable by any other
specific diagnosis. A biopsy is always required to reach a histological
diagnosis and to exclude malignancy. Regular review and often
repeated biopsy is required when the initial biopsy is negative for
malignancy. It is considered that patches of leucoplakia with a slightly
speckled appearance, with an associated erythroplasia or with
associated candidal hyphae have the greatest premalignant potential.
The example above shows an area of leucoplakia on the buccal
reflection of the lower jaw. The slightly red appearance surrounding
this lesion increases the possibility for malignant transformation.

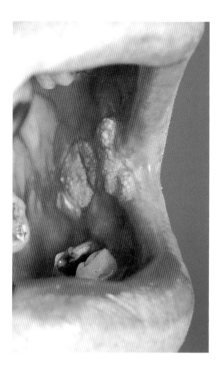

Figure 3.45
Leucoplakia (speckled)

The two areas of leucoplakia on the buccal mucosa of this patient have a slightly speckled appearance, which is associated with an increased potential for malignant transformation.

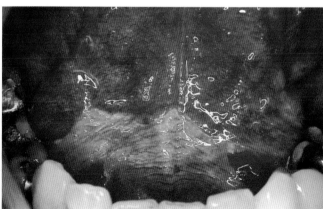

Figure 3.46
Leucoplakia (sublingual)

A full examination of all areas of the oral cavity is always required. Note the extensive area of leucoplakia that was 'hidden' on the undersurface of the tongue.

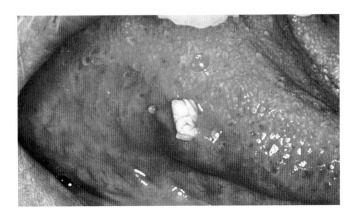

Figure 3.47
Leucoplakia (lingual keratosis)

A small, white keratotic papilloma can be seen on the lateral border of
this tongue. This was shown on histological examination to be a
severely dysplastic squamous papilloma. Surgical excision would
nearly always be appropriate for such a lesion.

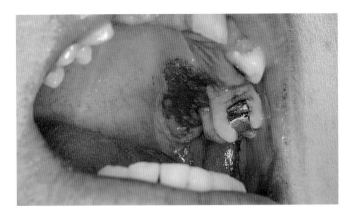

Figure 3.48
Erythroplakia (carcinoma in situ)

This patient had an area of leucoplakia visible on the hard palate,
which over a number of years developed a red appearance
('erythroplakia'). The malignant potential of erythroplakia is greater
than that of leucoplakia. The red ulcerative area seen on the hard
palate was found to be a carcinoma in situ at the latest biopsy.

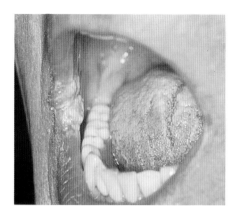

Figure 3.49
Leucoplakia (candidal)

The white heaped-up lesion at the corner of this mouth is an area of chronically hyperplastic epithelium infiltrated with candidal hyphae. The causal relationship between the leucoplakia and the candidal infection is unknown. These lesions are more likely to undergo malignant transformation than leucoplakia without Candida.

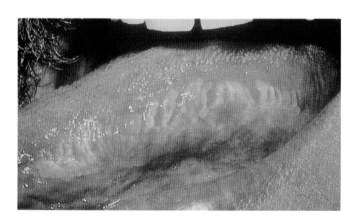

Figure 3.50
Leucoplakia (hairy leucoplakia)

Hairy leucoplakia is typically a white, slightly raised lesion with a corrugated surface. The lesion can be found throughout the oral cavity, but is most common along the lateral margins of the tongue and on the buccal surface of the cheek. The white ridged area shown along the lateral border of this tongue is hairy leucoplakia. Hairy leucoplakia is diagnostic of AIDS. The premalignant potential of hairy leucoplakia is at present uncertain.

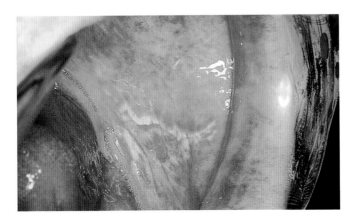

Figure 3.51
Lichen planus (non-erosive, buccal mucosa)

Lichen planus is a relatively common inflammatory disease of the oral mucous membranes, which may result either from local abnormalities of immune function or as a drug reaction. There is a wide range of appearances of lichen planus in the mouth ranging from a non-erosive variety through minor erosive to a major erosive type. This example is of a non–erosive lichen planus with its characteristic white lace-like reticulations.

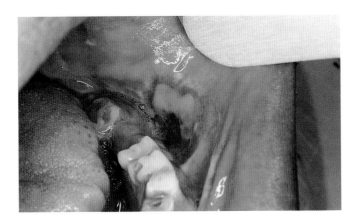

Figure 3.52
Lichen planus (minor erosive)

There has been a loss of the atrophic areas of the epithelium to form a shallow ulcer. The white reticulations can be seen surrounding the ulcer.

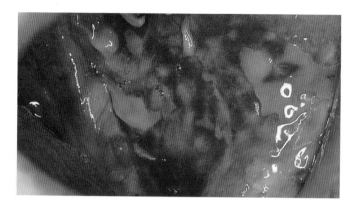

Figure 3.53
Lichen planus (major erosive)

In the major erosive variety of lichen planus, well-defined areas of extensive ulceration of sudden onset are characteristically seen on the buccal mucosa and along the lateral border of the tongue. No treatment is required for minor and non–erosive lichen planus, but major erosive lesions can be painful and require some intervention. Irritants to the mouth such as alcohol, tobacco, rough teeth and some drugs should be eliminated. Corticosteroids applied topically, intralesionally or systemically form the mainstay of treatment.

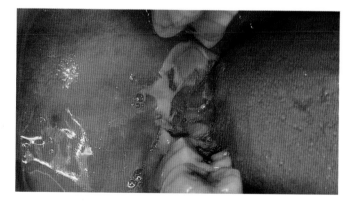

Figure 3.54
Aspirin burn (buccal sulcus)

One white but sometimes misdiagnosed condition of the mouth is an aspirin burn. The patient, as in this example, has pain in a tooth and holds an aspirin tablet next to the tooth in an effort to alleviate the ache. A white slough ulcer results.

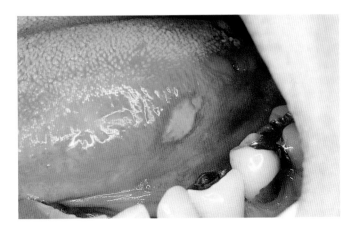

Figure 3.55
Aphthous stomatitis (aphthous ulcers) (canker sores)

Aphthous stomatitis is characterized by recurrent 'crops' of superficial ulcerations of the oral mucosa. The aetiology of this condition is unknown. These acute lesions are well demarcated with a yellow fibrin-covered base surrounded by a red halo. The white and extremely uncomfortable ulcer on the lateral border of this tongue is an aphthous ulcer. The characteristic erythematous surround to the ulcer is well demonstrated. Topical local anaesthetic sprays and gels are the mainstay of treatment. Judicious cautery to the base of the ulcer can, by deepening the lesion, relieve the pain, but it does increase the area that must heal.

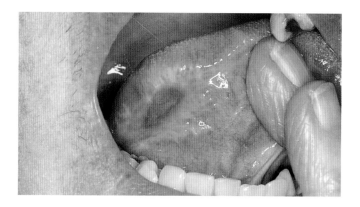

Figure 3.56
Solitary giant aphthous ulcer

The giant aphthous ulcer is usually bigger than the multiple aphthous ulcer and is, typically, greater than 1 cm in diameter. The red and large deep ulcer in the side of this patient's tongue is a giant aphthous ulcer. Pain was not particularly severe, owing to the full–thickness mucosal injury produced by the ulcer; however, this ulcer required several weeks to heal.

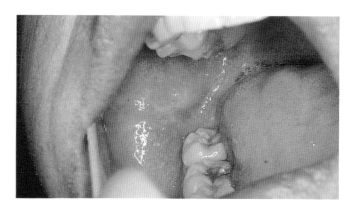

Figure 3.57
Cheek bite (traumatic factitious ulceration)

Some people, particularly those with a nervous disposition, chew the buccal mucosa with their molar teeth. This can result in an ulcer or more commonly a small white frictional area. The white area above the lower molar tooth in this illustration is the result of regular chewing of the buccal mucosa.

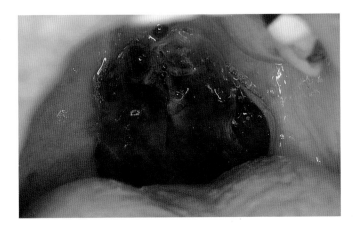

Figure 3.58
Pemphigus
Benign mucous membrane pemphigoid

Pemphigoid occurs in two principal forms: a predominantly cutaneous
form and a predominantly mucosal form. Subepithelial blisters develop
associated with the deposition of IgG class antibodies along the basal
zone. These oral bullae break down easily to leave large eroded areas,
particularly on the palate. Benign mucous membrane pemphigoid
represents a particular form of pemphigoid. The large bullae of benign
mucous membrane pemphigoid can be seen on this hard palate;
patients are rarely seen with this stage of the disease.

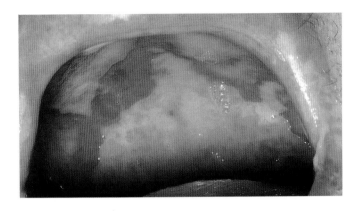

Figure 3.59
Benign mucous membrane pemphigoid

This illustration shows the more typical appearance of benign mucous membrane pemphigoid after the oral bullae have disintegrated leaving, particularly on the palate, large eroded areas. The erythematous areas are the pemphigoid.

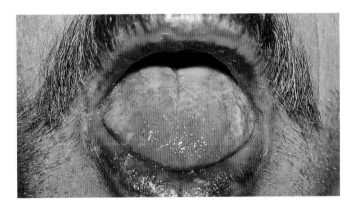

Figure 3.60
Stevens–Johnson syndrome (erythema multiforme)

Stevens–Johnson syndrome is an immunologically mediated syndrome comprising the triad of cutaneous lesions (erythema multiforme), stomatitis and conjunctivitis. This illustration shows the typical crusted, swollen and haemorrhagic appearance of the lips in Stevens–Johnson syndrome. An intact vesicle is visible on the left side of the tongue. A patient with this condition should always have his renal function checked and the urine examined for blood.

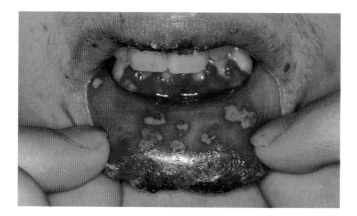

Figure 3.61
Herpetic gingivostomatitis

Herpetic gingivostomatitis is the gingival and oral response to a herpes
simplex infection. In this teenage patient the characteristic ulcers on the
lips and an intense painful inflammation of the gingivae can be seen.

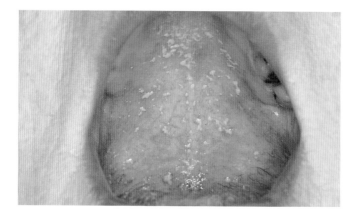

Figure 3.62
Candida

Candida species are effectively a commensal in the normal mouth. Any
loss of immunological competence can result in an acute
pseudomembranous candidiasis (thrush) of the mouth. There is,
however, a wide range of appearances to this condition. In this
illustration of mild thrush, a number of small white curds can be seen
on the hard palate.

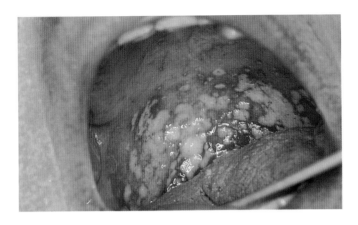

Figure 3.63
Candida

This illustration shows a more aggressive form of thrush with more extensive curd-like patches associated with an underlying painful erythema of the palate. It is worth remembering to treat the dentures as well as the mouth of a patient with candidiasis to avoid reinfection.

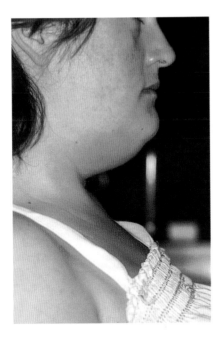

Figure 3.64
Ludwig's angina (floor of mouth cellulitis)

Ludwig's angina is an infection of the floor of the mouth, which results in cellulitis and swelling of the submandibular space. The floor of the mouth is extremely oedematous with posterosuperior elevation of the tongue. In this example the swelling is easily visible in the area under the chin, where there is also erythema that marks the extending cellulitis. Urgent hospital admission is required and emergency management of the airway can be required in severe cases.

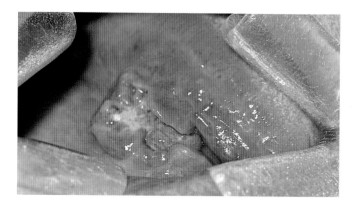

Figure 3.65
Squamous cell carcinoma (sublingual)

Squamous cell carcinoma may present in a number of shapes and sizes within the oral cavity: as an indurated ulcer, as a nodule or from an area of leucoplakia or erythroplakia. Any ulcer within the oral cavity that does not heal within 1 month should be biopsied to exclude malignancy. This example shows a sublingual/floor of mouth squamous cell carcinoma. Note the characteristic raised edges and the ulcerated central mass.

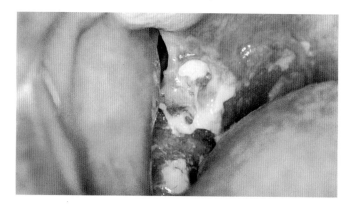

Figure 3.66
Squamous cell carcinoma (coffin corner)

There is an ulcerating and infiltrating squamous cell carcinoma developing behind the last lower molar tooth. This area is known as 'coffin corner' and is a site easily overlooked in clinical examination.

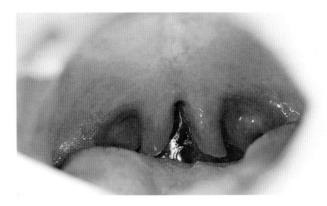

Figure 3.67
Bifid uvula

A bifid or cleft uvula is a minor congenital abnormality that may be associated with a submucosal separation of the soft palate (a submucosal cleft palate). Palpation along the midline of the soft palate is required to confirm the presence of the submucosal cleft.

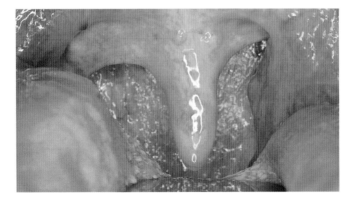

Figure 3.68
Long uvula

The normal length of the uvula is extremely varied. This example shows an elongated but normal uvula. In some instances, where the uvula becomes so long that it touches the laryngeal inlet and causes gagging or coughing, it may need to be excised.

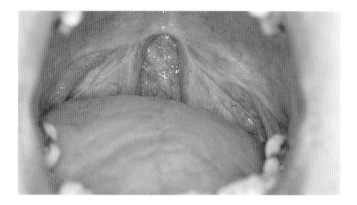

Figure 3.69
Uvulo-palatopharyngoplasty (UVPP)

A carbon dioxide laser has been used to excise the uvula and a central portion of the soft palate from the patient shown in this illustration. The procedure was effective in significantly reducing the sound volume of snoring produced by this patient. In current practice there are a number of different types of palatoplasty designed to reduce the intensity of snoring. There are, moreover, a number of different types of laser and types of surgical technique used to perform a palatoplasty.

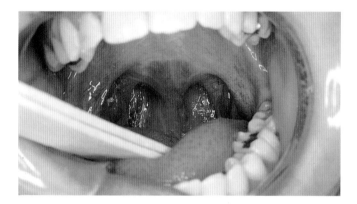

Figure 3.70
Palatoplasty

This patient has undergone a palatoplasty to relieve the velopharyngeal incompetence that resulted from a posterior cleft of the palate. Note the flap of pharyngeal mucosa inserted into the free margin of the soft palate.

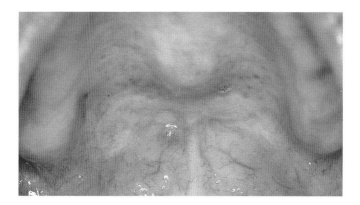

Figure 3.71
Torus palatinus

This discrete, hard, domed swelling in the midline of the hard palate is composed of compact lamellar bone; it is a torus palatinus. There is also a suspicious red raised nodule posterolateral to the torus palatinus. One can see a small palatal blood vessel almost pointing at the lesion. Excision biopsy demonstrated a small pleomorphic salivary adenoma.

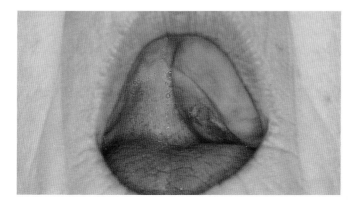

Figure 3.72
Ossifying fibroma

The hard, smooth lesion on the left half of this hard palate is an example of an ossifying fibroma. This lesion has been present and unchanged for many years; however, a recent biopsy site is visible.

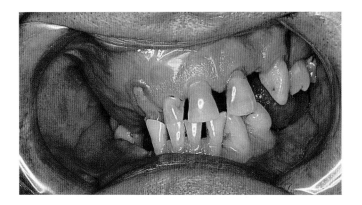

Figure 3.73
Fibrous dysplasia (dental bite alteration)

Fibrous dysplasia is a disease of unknown aetiology in which the
medullary cavity of the bone is replaced by fibrous tissue with a
potential for metaplastic new bone formation. In this example the
fibrous dysplasia has affected the maxilla and a gross abnormality of
the dental bite has developed.

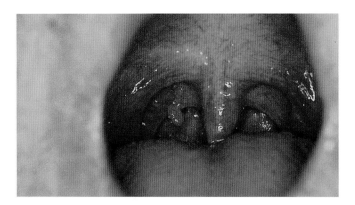

Figure 3.74
Papilloma (soft palate)

Oral papillomas are benign neoplasms derived from squamous
epithelium, which can be found in any part of the oral cavity,
although the soft palate, uvula and tonsillar regions are the most
common. The lesion can be broad–based or pedunculated and often,
but not always, has a cauliflower-like appearance. In this example the
papilloma arises from the right soft palate.

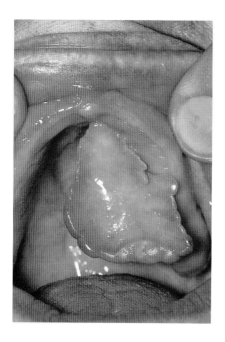

Figure 3.75
Fibroma of the palate

A palatal fibroma or similar lesion can sometimes be 'tucked' away from sight under a denture. In this illustration such a lesion is revealed and shown dangling by its stalk.

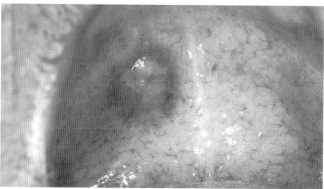

Figure 3.76
Pleomorphic adenoma

A pleomorphic adenoma can arise in any salivary gland. In this example a pleomorphic adenoma has arisen in a minor salivary gland situated in the hard palate. A single lobulated adenoma is more common than a multilobulated tumour on the palate. The red raised lesion on the hard palate is the pleomorphic adenoma. This adenoma has been repeatedly compressed by a denture plate. A fine-needle aspiration biopsy can confirm the diagnosis.

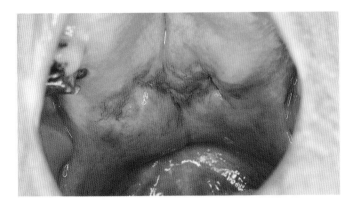

Figure 3.77
Lymphoma

An irregular, enlarging area of the palate raises a suspicion of
malignancy. The diffuse, infiltrative but non-ulcerative irregularity of
the centre of this hard palate was found to be a lymphoma on biopsy.
The tonsil is the most common site of oral lymphoma.

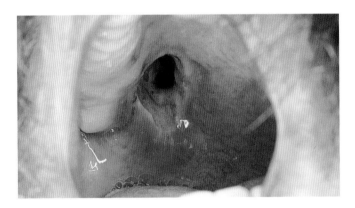

Figure 3.78
Adenocarcinoma

Adenocarcinoma within the oral cavity is a rare lesion, and
consequently the possibility that such a lesion is a secondary should
always be considered. Both squamous cell carcinoma and
adenocarcinoma in the region of the palate can produce a penetrative
ulcer and fistula between the mouth and the paranasal cavities at an
early stage. Adenocarcinoma created the palatal ulcer shown here.

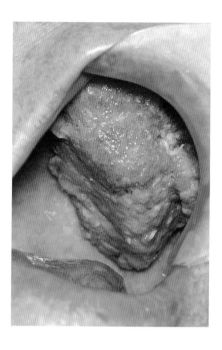

Figure 3.79
Verrucous carcinoma

A verrucous carcinoma typically (as shown in this illustration) has a pink, warty and non-ulcerated surface. It is a relatively soft tumour that characteristically occurs in those areas of the mouth where a tobacco chewing quid is regularly held. The diagnosis of a verrucous carcinoma is a combined clinical and histological diagnosis. This verrucous tumour extended from the buccal mucosa on to the hard palate.

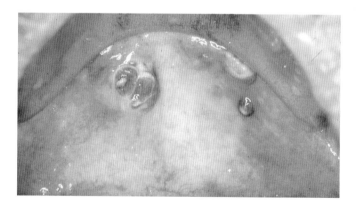

Figure 3.80
Kaposi's sarcoma

Each of the raised, bluish lesions on the hard palate of this patient, who has AIDS, is a Kaposi's sarcoma. The cutaneous lesions have a similar appearance. Kaposi's sarcoma is commonly associated with AIDS.

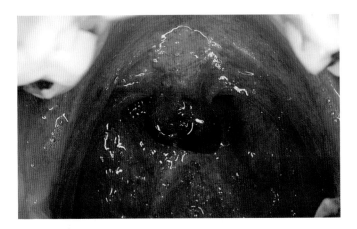

Figure 3.81
Blood blisters (spontaneous haematoma uvula)

Blood blisters (angina bullosa haemorrhagica) can arise within the
mouth as a result of trauma, clotting disorders or 'spontaneously'.
They often develop when a patient is eating and characteristically
occur on the hard or soft palate. In this example a spontaneous
haematoma of the uvula is visible. Simple rupture is usually curative.

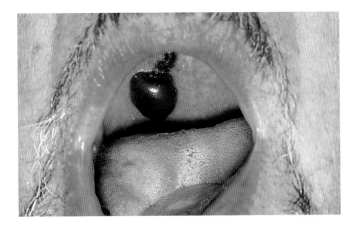

Figure 3.82
Palatal haematoma

The mucosa of the hard palate can be stripped into a small
haematoma or blood blister following very 'insignificant' trauma.
Rupture of the blister is curative.

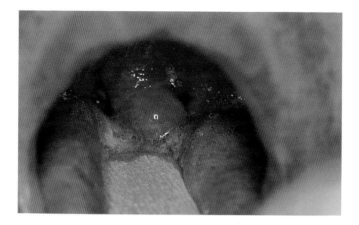

Figure 3.83
Acute oedema of the uvula

Acute swelling of the uvula may arise from trauma, as part of an
allergic reaction or as part of an infective process. In this example a
clumsy endotracheal intubation resulted in a swollen uvula. The
patient had the sensation of a 'lump in the back of the throat'; the
swelling resolved spontaneously within 72 hours. On occasion such an
oedematous uvula may continue to act like a pharyngeal foreign body,
causing the patient to gag constantly; an emergency resection of the
swollen uvula would be curative.

Tongue

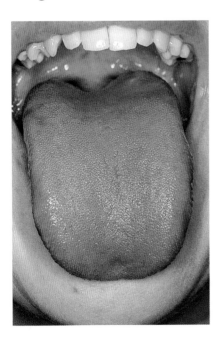

Figure 3.84
Normal tongue

The normal tongue, as it is protruded in the consulting room, has many shapes and sizes. This illustration shows a healthy normal tongue.

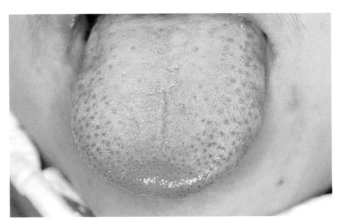

Figure 3.85
Normal tongue (dappled)

This illustration shows a mildly coated tongue with protrusion of papillae through the coating. This is a dappled tongue and also a normal finding.

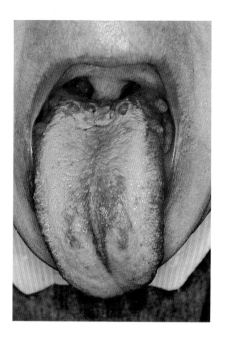

Figure 3.86
Coated tongue

A coated tongue may arise from dehydration, uraemia, prolonged use of oral antibiotics, cigarette smoking, persistent mouth breathing, poor oral hygiene or for no identifiable reason. This patient was a very heavy cigarette smoker, which was responsible for the thick coating on his tongue. Note the unsightly but not pathological red prominence of the circumvallate papillae appearing through the coated tongue.

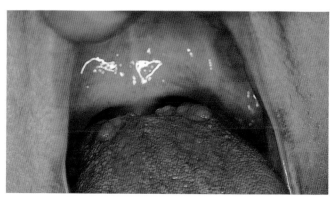

Figure 3.87
Prominent circumvallate papillae

Prominent circumvallate papillae can be a source of concern to a patient if they discover what they think is a suspicious swelling at the base of the tongue. This illustration shows how prominent circumvallate papillae can appear as a small red ridge, raised up on both sides of the base of the tongue. The characteristic apex to the V of the papillae is placed posteriorly on the tongue. Reassurance is all that is required.

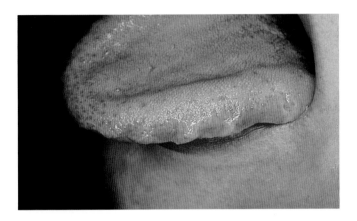

Figure 3.88
Crenellated tongue

The scalloped indentation seen along the lateral border of this
individual's relatively large tongue is a normal variant.

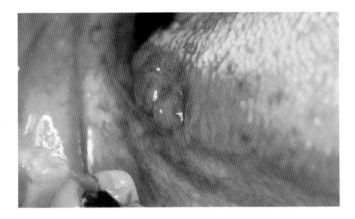

Figure 3.89
Lingual tonsils (lateral lymphoid tissue)

Lymphoid tissue within the base of the tongue is normal but often not
easily visible. Rarely, chronic infection may develop in this pad of
lingual lymphoid tissue. Prominent lymphoid tissue can sometimes be
seen protruding from the lateral base of the tongue. The lymphoid
tissue is the lobulated tissue on the right posterior lateral border of
the tongue. This tissue was an extension of the lymphoid tissue at the
base of the tongue (lingual tonsils).

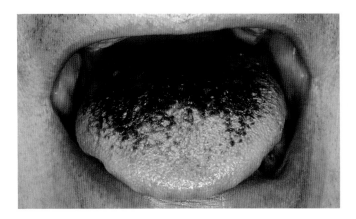

Figure 3.90
Black hairy tongue

This illustration shows a black hairy tongue. Filiform papillae elongate
to produce the 'hairy' coating. The true reason for the black colour
has never been explained, although antibiotics, tobacco, mouthwashes
and chromogenic bacteria have all been suspected. Cleaning the
tongue with a soft toothbrush or a 'tongue scraper' can be of help.

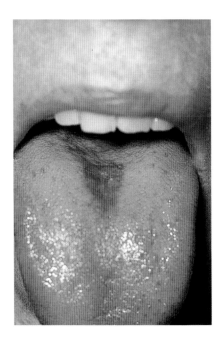

Figure 3.91
Median rhomboid glossitis

Median rhomboid glossitis
has been considered a
developmental abnormality
for a number of years;
however, recent work
suggests that this condition
arises from a mild local
candidal infection and that
'tongue clicking' against the
hard palate may be a
significant aetiological
factor. In this example, the
typically smooth, red,
diamond-shaped area
located centrally
immediately in front of the
circumvallate papillae can
be seen. Treatment is
usually not required.

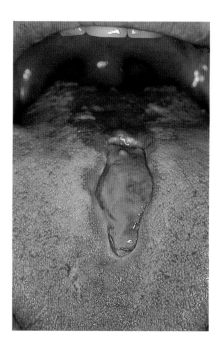

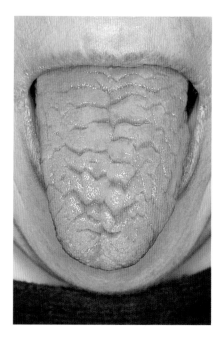

Figure 3.92
Median rhomboid glossitis

This unusual and severe example of
median rhomboid glossitis shows a
more extensive and almost ulcerated
defect located centrally immediately
in front of the circumvallate papillae.

Figure 3.93
Fissured tongue (scrotal tongue)

Almost 5% of the population have a
tongue with abnormal fissures and
grooves. The fissure pattern is
variable. Fissures tend to appear in
late childhood and deepen with age.
This illustration shows a tongue with
transverse fissures and one can
understand why the term 'scrotal
tongue' is occasionally used.

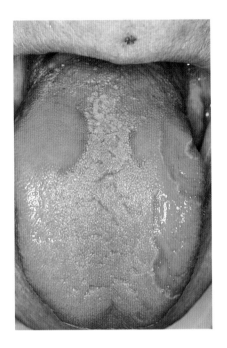 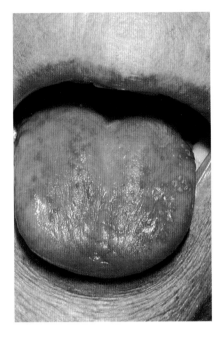

Figure 3.94
Geographic tongue (map tongue)

In some patients the filiform papillae disappear from localized areas of the tongue resulting in patchy red areas of depapillation, which is known as 'geographic tongue' or 'map tongue'. These patches repapillate after a variable time period and new areas of depapillation may occur on the tongue. Two large islands of depapillation on the lateral borders of the tongue are shown in this illustration. No treatment is required.

Figure 3.95
Atrophic glossitis

A beefy–red glazed tongue of iron deficiency is shown in this illustration. The smooth red surface develops as a result of the loss of the filiform papillae. Dysphagia from a web of the upper oesophagus can occur in association with an iron deficiency anaemia.

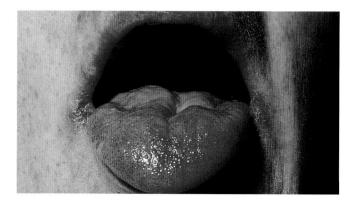

Figure 3.96
Atrophic glossitis and angular cheilitis

In this example an angular cheilitis can be seen in association with a
beefy–red glazed tongue of iron deficiency.

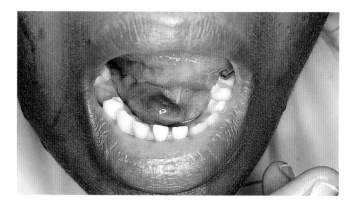

Figure 3.97
Ranula (mucocele of floor of mouth)

A ranula is a mucocele of the floor of the mouth, which may arise
from obstruction to the duct of one of the minor sublingual salivary
glands. This type of mucocele tends to be smaller and more
superficially placed. Ranulae may also arise from the sublingual
glands, and these ranulae tend to be larger and more deeply situated.
The blue discoloured swelling under the tongue on the floor of this
mouth is a ranula. Surgery is the treatment of choice for a ranula,
although recurrence is always a possibility.

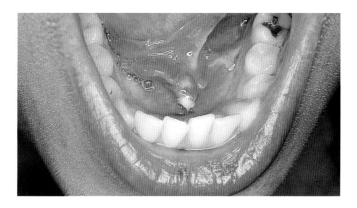

Figure 3.98
Submandibular duct stone

A submandibular duct stone is composed principally of calcium phosphate and develops around debris that collects in the submandibular ducts. In this illustration there is a terminal swelling within the submandibular duct and one can see a stone extruding from the duct.

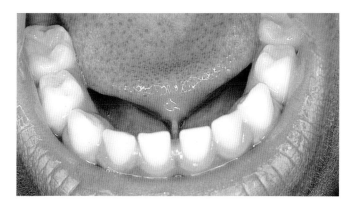

Figure 3.99
Tongue tie (ankyloglossia)

The frenulum of the tongue in this patient is abnormally short, resulting in an inability to protrude the tongue. This is known as a 'tongue tie'. No treatment is required, although release of the tongue tie is sometimes performed for socially cosmetic reasons. The division of the frenulum is a relatively simple procedure performed under local anaesthetic in adults but sometimes requiring a general anaesthetic in a child.

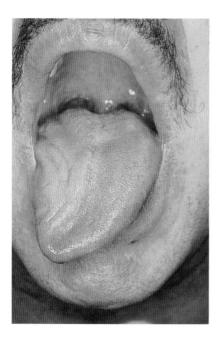

Figure 3.100
Hypoglossal nerve palsy

The right hypoglossal nerve of this patient was damaged in an accident. There is atrophy of the muscle bulk on the right side of the tongue and when the patient protrudes the tongue it deviates to the right (the side of the lesion).

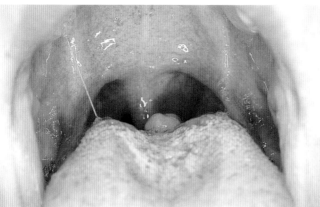

Figure 3.101
Lingual thyroid

The pink dome–shaped mass arising from the posterior surface of this patient's tongue is a lingual thyroid. A lingual thyroid is more liable to spontaneous internal haemorrhage than the normal thyroid gland. Significant expansion of a lingual thyroid can occur at puberty and in pregnancy. Occasionally, lingual thyroid can be the only functioning thyroid tissue in the body.

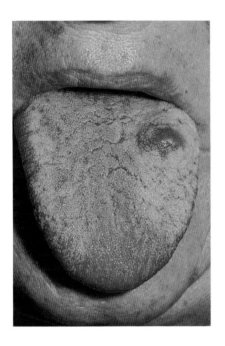

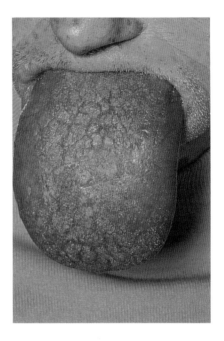

Figure 3.102
Haemangioma of tongue

The raised, blue, compressible lesion on the dorsum of this tongue has the characteristic features of a benign haemangioma. Surgical excision may be advised if haemorrhage is a problem.

Figure 3.103
Macroglossia (associated with Down's syndrome)

John Langdon Haydon Down, when describing 'congenital Mongolian idiots', identified a long, thickened and much roughened tongue as a characteristic feature. The enlargement of the tongue has been debated over the years, although the feature of protrusion beyond the lips is accepted. In this patient with Down's syndrome episodic massive enlargement of the tongue occurred. At postmortem examination a congenital lymphangiectasia of the tongue was found. The death was not caused by, or related to, the enlargement of the tongue.

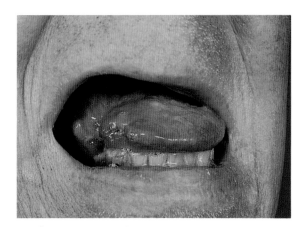

Figure 3.104
Squamous cell carcinoma of the tongue

Squamous cell carcinoma of the tongue can present as an ulcer, a
nodule or simply an area of induration of the tongue. In this patient
there is a characteristic ulcerative, infiltrative and advanced squamous
cell carcinoma of the lateral border of the tongue, which caused severe
limitation of tongue movement. Treatment of such a tumour may
involve surgery and/or radiotherapy.

Oropharynx

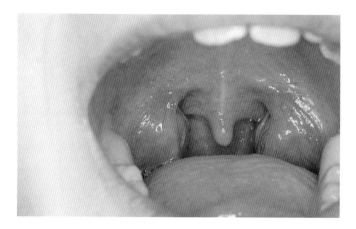

Figure 3.105
Normal tonsils

The appearance of the normal palatine tonsils is extremely varied. The tonsils may appear to protrude so far that they almost meet in the midline or they may be buried in the oropharyngeal wall to such an extent that only the tip of the tonsil is visible. This example shows a pair of normal tonsils placed approximately in the mid range of tonsil protrusion. The extent of protrusion into the oropharynx does not correlate with the overall size of the palatine tonsil.

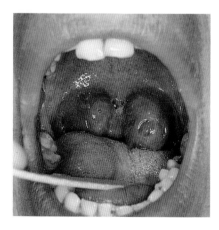

Figure 3.106
Obstructive tonsils

This patient has very large tonsils, which almost meet in the midline. Occasionally the use of a tongue depressor can provoke a gag reflex when examining the palatine tonsils. A gag reflex can cause the palatine tonsils to be pushed towards the midline thus giving a false appearance of 'enlarged tonsils'. This patient did not gag as this picture was taken! Tonsillectomy is curative of obstructive tonsils.

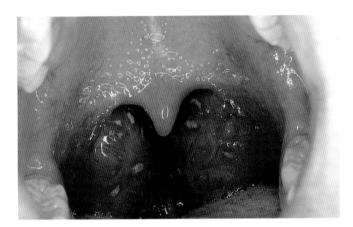

Figure 3.107
Acute tonsillitis (recurrent tonsillitis)

The beta-haemolytic streptococcus is the most common bacterium
cultured from the throat swab of a patient with acute bacterial
tonsillitis. This illustration shows the follicular variety of acute tonsillitis.
There is no characteristic clinical appearance of the palatine tonsils that
will either confirm or refute the diagnosis of recurrent episodes of acute
tonsillitis (recurrent acute tonsillitis). Some clinicians consider the
presence of erythema of the anterior pillar to be of diagnostic
significance; the history, however, is the most important feature in the
diagnosis of acute recurrent tonsillitis.

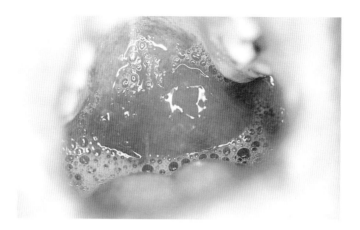

Figure 3.108
Peritonsillar abscess (quinsy)

A peritonsillar abscess is a bacterial abscess located between the tonsillar capsule and the lateral pharyngeal wall. Marked trismus is commonly present. In this illustration, oedema around the affected left tonsil stretches on to the palate and local retention of saliva can be seen. The abscess is not yet 'pointing'. Trismus makes the photography of a peritonsillar abscess difficult. Treatment requires needle aspiration or incision and drainage combined with antibiotic therapy.

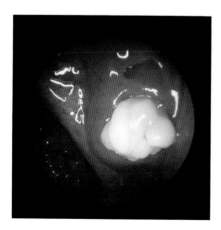

Figure 3.109
Tonsil crypt with debris (chronic cryptic tonsillitis)

Tonsillar crypts can collect debris, as shown in this endoscopically produced illustration. Some patients can become quite adept at manually expressing the debris from their crypts. Excessive collection of debris in multiple crypts may be the cause of halitosis.

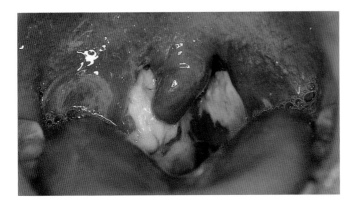

Figure 3.110
Infectious mononucleosis (glandular fever)

Acutely swollen and juicy-looking tonsils covered with yellow debris and often associated with palatal petechiae are characteristic of infectious mononucleosis (glandular fever). Despite their swollen and juicy appearance, the tonsils were extremely hard and caused considerable discomfort in swallowing. Oral steroids were used to alleviate some of the tonsillar swelling and as a consequence relieve the pain of swallowing.

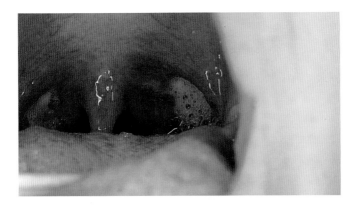

Figure 3.111
Normal postoperative tonsillectomy bed after 1 week

One week after an elective tonsillectomy, some pooling of saliva in the tonsil bed is still present. If the saliva is cleared, the base of the tonsil bed usually contains a whitish–grey slough.

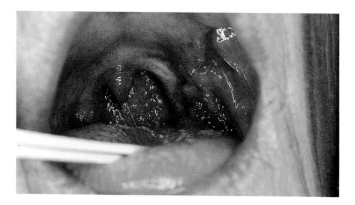

Figure 3.112
Squamous cell carcinoma of tonsil

The ulcerated and indurated lesion of the left tonsil bed is a squamous cell carcinoma. Such lesions sometimes spread to the tonsil from the retromolar trigone or 'coffin corner'. A biopsy to confirm the diagnosis followed by an extensive endoscopic and CT assessment of the upper aerodigestive tract is required prior to definitive treatment. Treatment may require radiotherapy combined with surgical excision of the lesion. A reconstruction with a myocutaneous or free flap may be needed to close the surgical defect and retain satisfactory oral function.

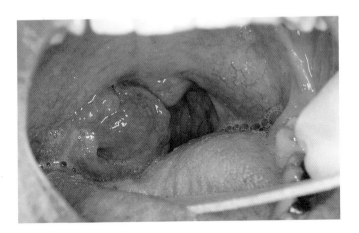

Figure 3.113
Lymphoma of tonsil

This large fleshy swelling of the right palatine tonsil is characteristic of lymphoma. This was a non-Hodgkin's lymphoma. A unilateral tonsillar swelling should be excised urgently and examined by histology to exclude malignancy.

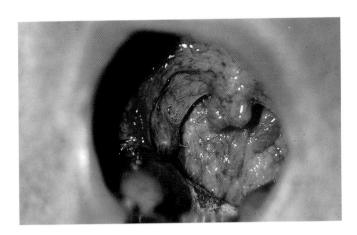

Figure 3.114
Fish bone in tonsil

This patient who ate improperly boned fish presented with a fishbone impacted in the left tonsil. If a suspected fishbone cannot be found, then plain radiography of the suspected area can be helpful. A radiolucent fishbone can produce an identifiable 'air indentation' on the X-ray.

4 The larynx

Direct visual inspection of the larynx and hypopharynx is not possible without a general anaesthetic or a significant degree of sedation and topical anaesthesia. Competent examination of the pharynx and larynx, in an awake patient, requires indirect laryngoscopy, which may be performed with a laryngeal mirror, flexible fibreoptic laryngoscope or a rigid-rod angled telescope.

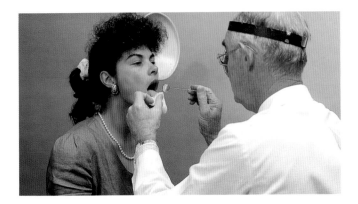

Figure 4.1
Laryngeal mirror

Indirect laryngoscopy using a circular laryngeal mirror and reflected light has been the traditional method of laryngeal examination. The equipment is inexpensive and can give a very satisfactory view of the larynx and pharynx. This technique, however, requires a moderate level of skill and training. The use of topical anaesthesia is occasionally required in those patients who have a strong gag reflex.

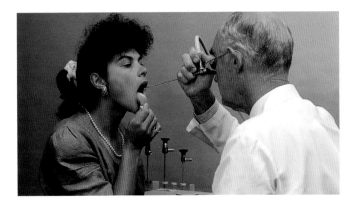

Figure 4.2
Laryngeal telescope

Indirect laryngoscopy using a rigid, 4.0 mm diameter 70° angled Hopkins rod lens laryngeal telescope can provide a very clear view of the larynx, the laryngopharynx and the base of the tongue.

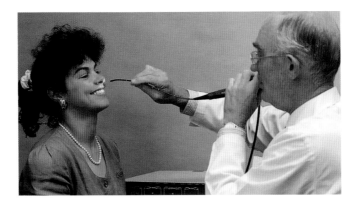

Figure 4.3
Flexible nasopharyngolaryngoscope

A flexible nasopharyngolaryngoscope, of 3.5 mm diameter, can easily
be passed through one nasal cavity which has been adequately
prepared with topical anaesthesia and decongestant spray. Whilst the
view of the larynx is not as sharp and clear as that provided by the
mirror or rigid telescope, the ease of use and the mobility of the
flexible nasopharyngolaryngoscope make it a good instrument for
examination of the upper airway.

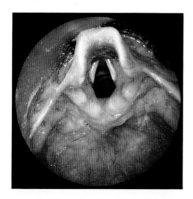

Figure 4.4
Three views of child's normal larynx

One cannot examine all areas of the larynx at once, as demonstrated with these three views. The examiner must therefore mentally construct a composite picture. The first view shows an overall view of the laryngopharynx, the second the supraglottic structures, and third the glottis, subglottis and upper trachea.

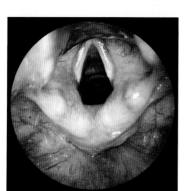

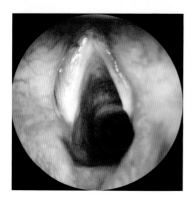

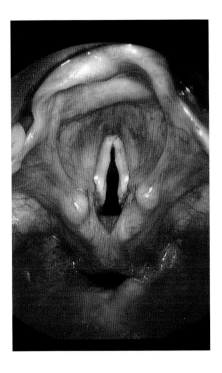

Figure 4.5
Larynx and hypopharynx

The Lindholm laryngoscope gives an excellent panoramic view of the supraglottic and glottic structures and, in this case, the postcricoid region is also widely exposed.

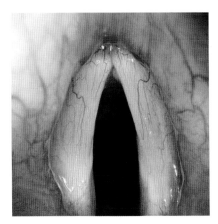

Figure 4.6
Vocal folds

This illustration shows the anterior commissure (the anterior angle between the right and left true vocal cords) and the false cords in a normal adult.

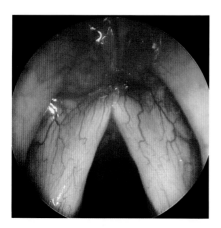

Figure 4.7
Close-up of anterior commissure

The anterior commissure can be a 'hidden' area to direct inspection. The anterior commissure and the 'hidden' area above it are clearly seen with a 30° laryngeal telescope.

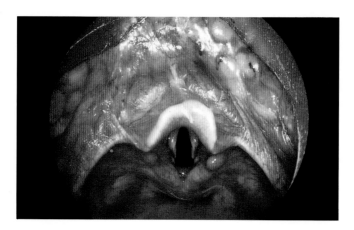

Figure 4.8
Base of tongue

This illustration shows the base of the tongue, valleculae, glosso-epiglottic fold, epiglottis and glossopharyngeal folds. This view was obtained with a Lindholm laryngoscope positioned at the base of the tongue.

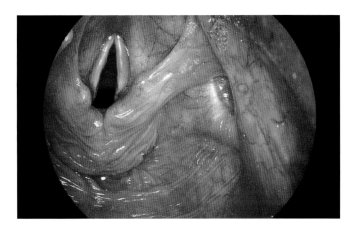

Figure 4.9
Laryngopharynx

By angling the Lindholm laryngoscope, the lateral pharyngeal wall,
piriform fossa and part of the postcricoid region can be demonstrated.

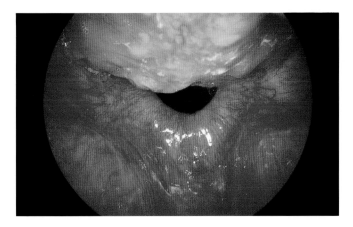

Figure 4.10
Postcricoid region

The postcricoid region and cricopharyngeus muscle have been exposed
with the Lindholm laryngoscope.

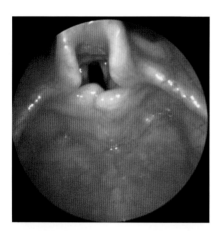

Figure 4.11
Laryngomalacia

Laryngomalacia ('floppy larynx') is the most common cause of laryngeal stridor in infants. As inspiration commences there is partial inward collapse of the supraglottic structures, the epiglottis curls upon itself and the cuneiform cartilages are sucked into the glottic opening. At maximum inspiration there is only a small supraglottic laryngeal opening. During expiration the airway is unimpeded. These serial photographs illustrate the problem.

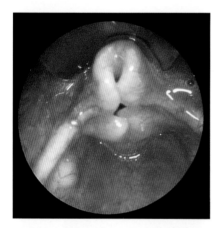

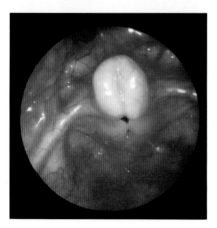

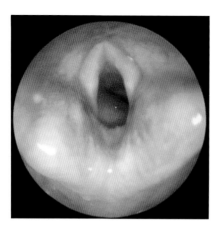

Figure 4.12
Subglottic haemangioma

This left subglottic haemangioma extends into the posterior subglottic space. Congenital subglottic haemangiomas are associated with large or small facial or neck haemangiomas in about 50% of cases. Biopsy is necessary only when the diagnosis is in doubt.

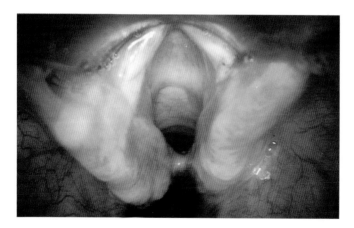

Figure 4.13
Congenital posterior laryngeal cleft

This illustration demonstrates a posterior laryngeal cleft extending into the cricoid cartilage. It is typical that, endoscopically, the upper oesophageal lumen can be seen. Persistent aspiration during feeding is the cardinal feature of a congenital posterior laryngeal cleft.

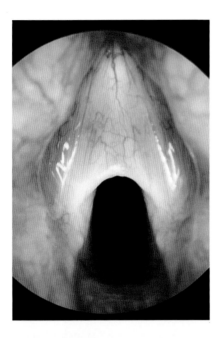

Figure 4.14
Medium–sized congenital glottic web

This baby had a husky cry but no airway obstruction. Note the medium-sized, moderately thick congenital anterior glottic web. Most congenital webs are anteriorly placed.

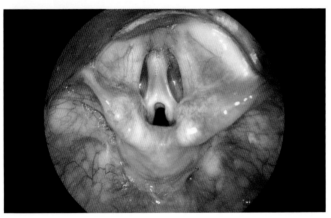

Figure 4.15
Large congenital glottic web

This patient has a large congenital glottic web. The vocal ligaments can be seen and the laryngeal ventricles are prominent. There was an associated thick subglottic stenosis about 12–15 mm in length. Severe airway obstruction at birth required a tracheotomy; the lesion was surgically repaired at 4.5 years of age.

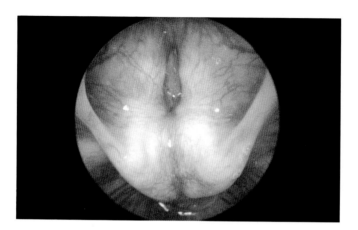

Figure 4.16
Laryngeal atresia

Attempted intubation at birth was unsuccessful in this newborn with laryngeal atresia. Life was maintained for about 20 minutes by positive pressure ventilation via an H-type tracheo-oesophageal fistula until an emergency tracheotomy was performed.

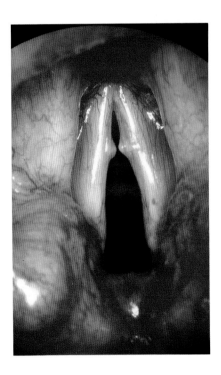

Figure 4.17
Vocal nodules

Vocal nodules occur in both adults and children (mostly boys). They vary in colour, contour and size and are usually similar on each side. These nodules characteristically occur at the junction of the anterior third and the posterior two–thirds of the vocal cords. Histological examination of vocal nodules shows thickened epithelium, submucosal oedema, microcystic degeneration and hyalinization in Reinke's space. Voice therapy may be beneficial, but when the nodules cause troublesome hoarseness for months or years microsurgical removal may be considered. These are the vocal nodules of a 12-year-old boy who presented with chronic intermittent huskiness unresponsive to speech therapy.

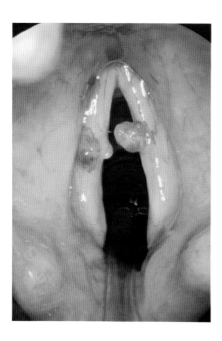

Figure 4.18
Vocal nodules

The unusual appearance of these vocal nodules is apparently due to degeneration within the vocal nodules of a woman in her thirties who had refused treatment for many years.

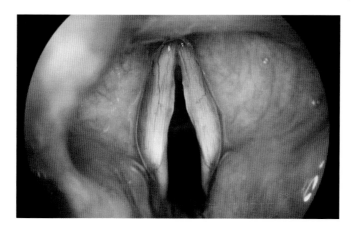

Figure 4.19
Vocal nodules (chronic laryngitis)

Vocal nodules often have a prominent fusiform longitudinal swelling. In this case, however, there is no focal nodular abnormality and consequently the term 'vocal nodules' would be a misnomer.

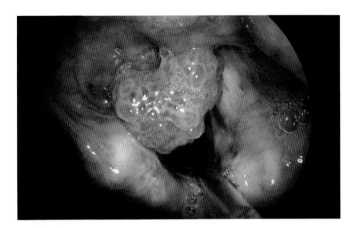

Figure 4.20
Laryngeal papillomatosis (supraglottic)

Papillomas, caused by the human papillomavirus, occur in the upper airway in patients of any age, about two-thirds being younger than 15 years. The highest incidence is before the age of 5 years. Papillomas occur most commonly in the larynx, but may be found elsewhere in the upper respiratory tract from the nasal mucosa to the lung parenchyma and even in the oesophagus. The large papillomatous mass in a left supraglottic larynx had a relatively small pedicle, which allowed excision of the mass with a carbon dioxide laser.

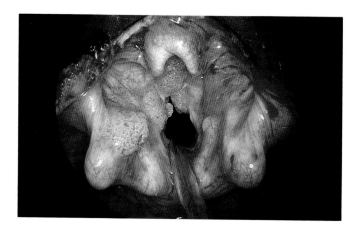

Figure 4.21
Laryngeal papillomatosis (widespread)

There is no interrelationship between puberty and the age at onset,
the rate of control or the rate of recurrence. Consequently, any patient
should be treated without regard to his or her age since there is no
tendency for regression at puberty. Although unexpected remissions do
occur, this disease is notorious for frequent recurrences and multiple
sites of involvement. This overall view of the larynx shows many
deposits of papilloma. No normal vocal folds can be seen.

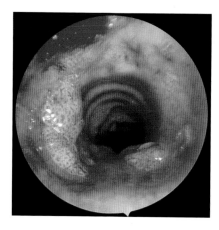

Figure 4.22
Respiratory
papillomatosis

This patient has developed
multiple areas of papilloma
in the upper and lower
trachea. Patients who have
aggressively growing lesions
in the trachea or bronchi
may develop papillomatous
nodules in the lung
parenchyma. They should
have a chest radiograph or
CT scan to assess the
status of their lungs.

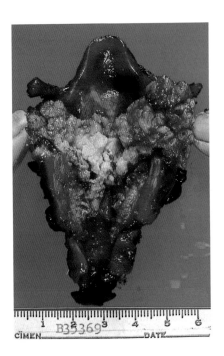

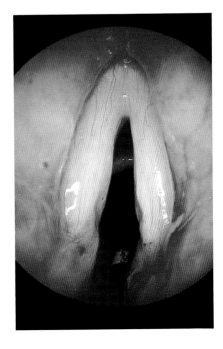

Figure 4.23
Respiratory papillomatosis
(verrucous carcinoma)

Laryngeal papillomas may undergo
malignant degeneration. This
laryngectomy specimen is from a 15-
year-old boy who had a tracheotomy
at the age of 7 years and was
advised to return 'after puberty'.
Histological examination showed that
a verrucous carcinoma had
developed.

Figure 4.24
Reinke's oedema

Reinke's oedema occurs when excess
fluid accumulates in Reinke's space.
Chronic oedema in Reinke's space
may be unilateral or bilateral and
can progress to the formation of
large, bilateral oedematous vocal cord
polyps. Other polyps may be
fusiform, pedunculated or
generalized. Reinke's oedema results
in a hoarse, low-pitched voice.

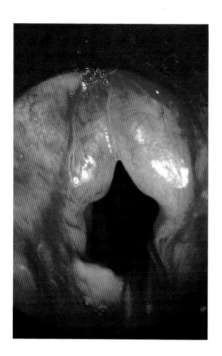

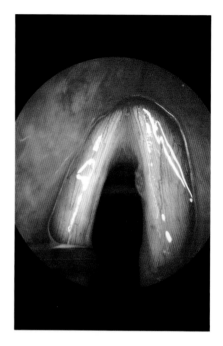

Figure 4.25
Reinke's oedema (severe)

Reinke's space is a potential space
between the surface mucosa of the
vocal fold and the medial
thyroarytenoid (vocalis) muscle and
vocal ligament. The space stretches
from the tip of the vocal process to
the anterior commissure, contains
loose areolar tissue and allows free
movement and vibration of the
mucosa of the vocal folds during
phonation. The severe bilateral
Reinke's oedema with bilateral
generalized polypoidal degeneration in
this patient was successfully treated
by staged microlaryngeal surgical
treatment (first one side and later the
other side).

Figure 4.26
Vocal cord polyp

There is a small, slightly irregular
polyp on the edge and undersurface
of the right vocal fold. Microsurgical
removal with cup forceps and
scissors gives a better result in this
type of polyp than the laser.

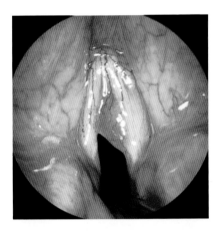

Figure 4.27
Vocal cord polyp

There is a large, thin-walled fusiform polyp of the right vocal fold. The vascular congestion, venous stasis and degree of oedema may vary with voice use.

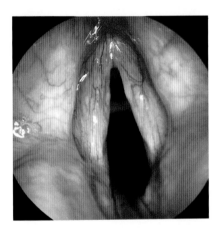

Figure 4.28
Chronic laryngitis

This male patient with chronic laryngitis had a hoarse, low-pitched voice. Note the irregular vocal fold edges, some oedema and the dilated blood vessels.

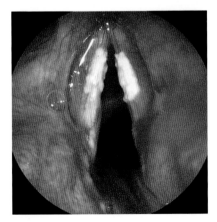

Figure 4.29
Chronic fungal laryngitis

The fungal laryngitis in this teenage boy was the result of the long-term inhalation of a metered aerosol synthetic steroid spray for the treatment of asthma.

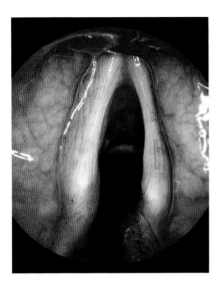

Figure 4.30
Presbyphonia

'Presbyphonia' is the term used to describe the degeneration that occurs in some patients with age. Presbyphonia is characterized by a visible bowing of the vocal folds with incomplete glottic closure causing a weak, breathy voice that tires with prolonged use. The flaccidity of the vocal folds slowly becomes worse with age.

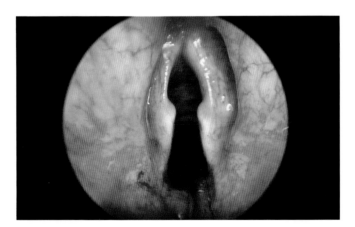

Figure 4.31
Presbyphonia

The advanced bowing of the vocal folds and the 'arrowhead' appearance of presbyphonia. These changes occur more commonly in men. Surgical procedures to increase the tension in the vocal folds appear to have promising short-term results. It appears that careful injection of collagen or fat may improve the voice.

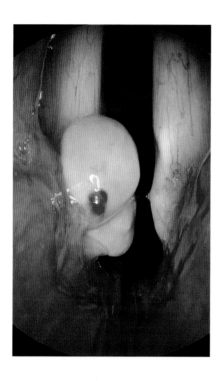

Figure 4.32
Vocal granuloma

Vocal granulomas are uncommon but readily recognized, rounded, sometimes bilobed or even multilobed, yellow, pink or pale–red opalescent masses arising from a pedicle on the posterior one-third of the vocal cord adjacent to the vocal process and medial surface of the arytenoid cartilage. Most patients have some degree of hoarseness but in others the voice may be near normal. There is often a feeling of irritation and a desire to clear the throat. Microlaryngoscopy and excision biopsy for histological examination will exclude malignancy or other specific granuloma. Specific granulomas such as tuberculosis, histoplasmosis, coccidioidomycosis, blastomycosis, syphilis, leprosy, sarcoidosis, Wegener's granulomatosis, scleroma and Crohn's disease may occur in the larynx on rare occasions.

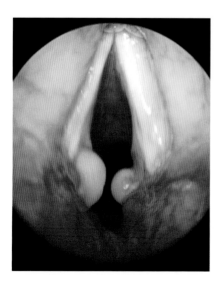

Figure 4.33
Bilateral intubation granulomas

This illustration demonstrates bilateral intubation granulomas larger on the left side than the right, found only a few weeks after prolonged intubation. The patient was intubated following severe smoke inhalation.

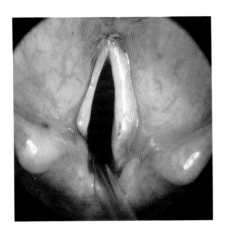 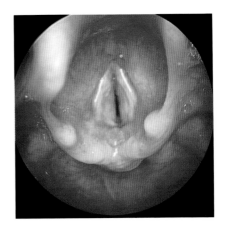

Figure 4.34
Vocal cord paralysis

Most vocal cord palsies are caused
by peripheral lesions of the recurrent
laryngeal nerve. The aetiology may be
post–thyroidectomy or other neck
surgery, malignancy (particularly lung
tumours), idiopathic, or external
trauma. The illustration shows a
long-standing left vocal cord paralysis
producing atrophy and shortening of
the left vocal cord.

Figure 4.35
Acute laryngotracheitis

Acute viral laryngotracheitis,
commonly known as 'croup', is much
more prevalent than acute
epiglottitis, and much less likely to
cause severe airway obstruction.
Croup and epiglottitis are usually
easy to distinguish. This example
shows marked narrowing of the
subglottic airway by inflammation
and oedematous swelling. Note the
absence of supraglottic swelling.

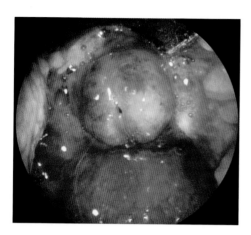

Figure 4.36
Acute epiglottitis

The epiglottis in acute epiglottitis is grossly swollen, often with a mottled yellow and red appearance. Intubation of this narrow and potentially obstructed airway requires experience and skill; an immediate emergency tracheostomy may occasionally be required. Acute epiglottitis is usually caused by *Haemophilus influenzae B*.

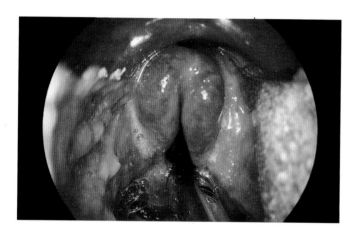

Figure 4.37
Acute epiglottitis after intubation

This patient had a 10-hour history of respiratory distress, quiet inspiratory stridor, muffled voice, painful swallowing and drooling of saliva. Endotracheal intubation is the treatment of choice to relieve the airway obstruction.

Laryngeal leucoplakia, dysplasia and neoplasia

'Dysplasia' is a histological term describing microscopic changes that indicate possible progression to malignancy. The characteristic cellular changes include atypical cells with large hyperchromatic nuclei and loss of cellular polarity. There is irregular stratification and increased mitosis. In carcinoma in situ (intraepithelial carcinoma) the basal membrane is preserved while in invasive carcinoma the nests or tongues of cells penetrate the basement membrane and infiltrate the deeper tissues. Most malignant laryngeal tumours are squamous cell carcinomas.

Leucoplakia is a white patch in the larynx without a histological diagnosis. Dysplastic epithelium is often white. Any area of leucoplakia or dysplastic epithelium within the larynx requires an urgent biopsy, usually under microlaryngeal control, to provide an accurate diagnosis.

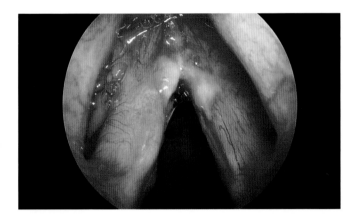

Figure 4.38
Leucoplakia

This illustration shows leucoplakia at the anterior commissure extending on to the right and left vocal folds. Biopsies revealed hyperkeratosis with atypia. Regular follow-up was required.

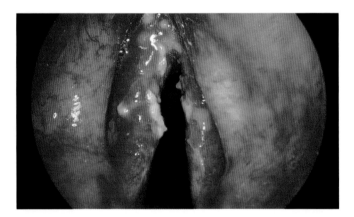

Figure 4.39
Severe dysplasia

This illustration shows extensive abnormality within both vocal folds: there are multiple areas of irregular leucoplakia and erythroplasia, and malignancy was suspected. The histological examination demonstrated severe hyperkeratosis and dysplasia. Regular review and repeat biopsy were required.

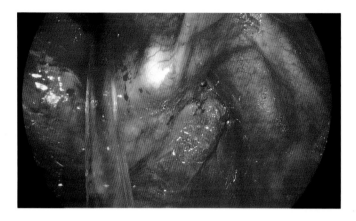

Figure 4.40
Carcinoma in situ

There is a raised lesion within an irregular surface in the right piriform fossa. The ventilatory catheter passes between the arytenoids (visible) and the vocal cords into the trachea. The lesion looks like a squamous cell carcinoma but the histology demonstrated a carcinoma in situ.

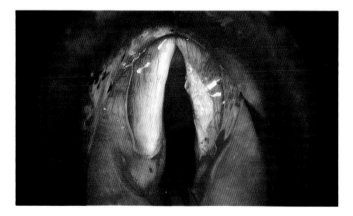

Figure 4.41
Squamous cell carcinoma

There is an irregular lesion of the central third of the right vocal cord which was shown to be an infiltrating squamous cell carcinoma. This lesion was effectively treated by laser excision with no recurrence 5 years later. In some countries this lesion would have been treated by radiotherapy.

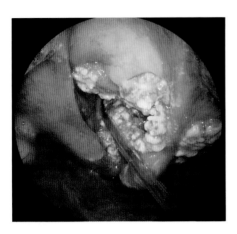

Figure 4.42
Squamous cell carcinoma

There is an infiltrating squamous
cell carcinoma of the supraglottic
larynx involving the tubercle of
the epiglottis, false vocal cord
and aryepiglottic fold and
ulcerating into the medial aspect
of the right piriform fossa. The
patient presented with a hoarse
voice and increasing stridor. A
laryngectomy was required.

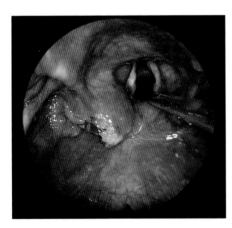

Figure 4.43
Squamous cell carcinoma

This illustration demonstrates an
infiltrating squamous cell
carcinoma involving the anterior
and lateral wall of the left
piriform fossa and the upper
aspect of the arytenoid. A tumour
of the pyriform fossa tends to
present late because it does not
produce hoarseness (there is no
arytenoid or vocal cord invasion)
and does not obstruct the airway
until the tumour is very large.
This squamous cell carcinoma
was treated with radiotherapy.

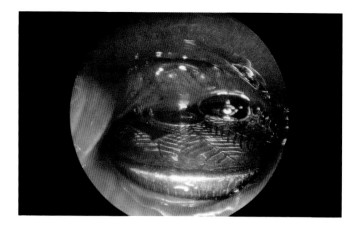

Figure 4.44
Ingested foreign body: coin

Sharp ingested foreign bodies such as fishbones may impact in the
tonsil, base of tongue, laryngopharynx or postcricoid region. Drawing
pins, badges and clasps usually impact in the upper oesophagus.
Pieces of meat, vegetables, fruit and coins are usually held up in the
upper oesophagus. A plain radiograph will show a radio-opaque
foreign body such as a coin or a piece of bone. This coin (Australian
10 cents) impacted in the upper oesophagus is shown immediately
before removal using a rigid oesophagoscope under general
anaesthetic.

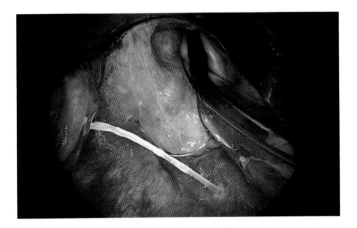

Figure 4.45
Ingested foreign body: fishbone

This large fishbone has impacted in the lateral pharyngeal wall, the sharp end medially in the posterior pharyngeal wall.

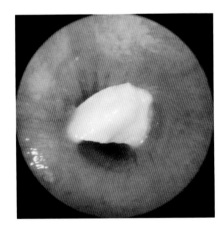

Figure 4.46
Inhaled foreign body: peanut

The highest incidence of inhaled foreign body is in the second and third years of life. There is usually a history of a sudden coughing attack, choking, gagging, gasping, wheezing and cyanosis lasting minutes or hours. The illustration shows a peanut fragment impacted in the left main bronchus just prior to endoscopic removal. There is little surrounding tissue reaction in the airway, but if the peanut remains there will be a considerable inflammatory reaction.

5 The neck

A systematic and thorough technique for the examination of the structures contained in the neck is imperative if abnormalities are not to be missed. Each individual practitioner should develop a standard systematic routine for examining all areas of the neck.

The neck should first be fully exposed to below the levels of the clavicles to facilitate a thorough examination of all areas. The initial inspection of the neck may reveal an obvious swelling, or the way in which the patient is 'holding' his or her head may suggest the presence of an inflammatory process. One technique of examination of the neck is described below.

The examination commences with an inspection of the neck from the front and from both sides. The practitioner then stands behind the seated patient. The patient is asked to relax and gently flex the neck forward while the examiner's fingers are placed simultaneously on each mastoid process. The fingers then palpate in turn the preauricular area and the surface of the parotid gland, return under the pinna to the postauricular sulcus and move to the occiput before returning to the mastoid process.

The fingers now palpate down the anterior border of the trapezius to the clavicle, traverse the supraclavicular fossa and ascend the posterior border of the sternomastoid before returning to the mastoid process.

The fingers then move down the anterior border of the sternomastoid to the sternal notch and ascend in the midline. Care is required during this manoeuvre to avoid excessive and bilateral palpation over the carotid bulbs as this may occasionally produce syncope.

As the fingers ascend in the midline, the thyroid gland is palpated. If the patient is asked to take a swallow at this time the movement of the thyroid gland can be assessed. The fingers progress in the midline to the point of the chin and palpate along the submental and submandibular triangles before returning to the mastoid process.

If there is a palpable or described abnormality in the submental or submandibular regions then bimanual palpation with a gloved finger inserted into the mouth is mandatory.

If a significant external abnormality is found on examination of the neck then a thorough examination of the oral cavity, pharynx and larynx is generally required.

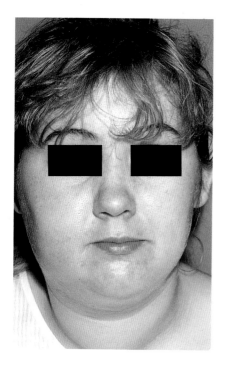

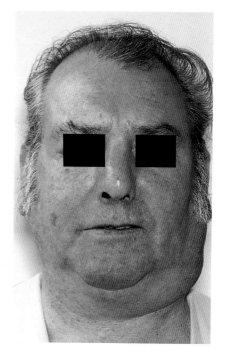

Figure 5.1
Viral parotitis (mumps)

Mumps is the most common cause of
acute parotitis. The mumps virus is a
member of the paramyxovirus group.
Swelling of one or both parotid
glands is common, with the swelling
located characteristically below and
in front of the ear. The swollen
parotid gland may push the earlobe
forward and laterally, and in severe
cases it may even limit jaw
movement. The swelling of one side
may precede the other by as much
as 4 days. This teenager has bilateral
parotid swellings as a result of
mumps.

Figure 5.2
Bacterial parotitis

Bacterial parotitis is most often due
to a staphylococcal infection of the
parotid gland in a dehydrated
patient. This situation can arise in
those patients with uncontrolled
diabetes, renal failure or severe
electrolyte disturbance. The gland
becomes acutely swollen and tender
and may, as shown in this case,
progress to frank abscess formation.
The skin overlying the gland has
become red as the abscess develops.

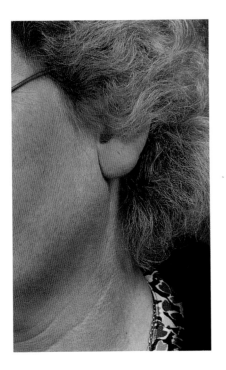

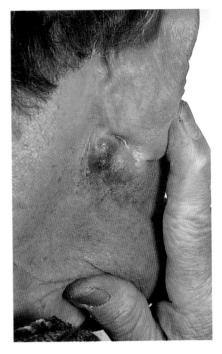

Figure 5.3
Parotid tumour (lymphoma)

A development of a rapidly swelling
and uncomfortable mass in the
parotid region is highly suspicious of
malignancy. This female patient had
a rapidly enlarging mass in the
parotid. Note how the earlobe is
pushed laterally. Histology showed
this mass to be a lymphoma. The
absence of a facial palsy in
association with rapidly expanding
parotid tumour suggests the presence
of a lymphomatous tumour. Fine-
needle aspiration cytology is often
helpful in establishing the diagnosis
of a parotid swelling. A pleomorphic
adenoma is the most common
tumour of the parotid gland.

Figure 5.4
**Parotid tumour (mucoepidermoid
carcinoma)**

This patient has a mass in the right
parotid gland which is beginning to
ulcerate through the skin below and
behind the ear. Cutaneous
breakthrough and subsequent
ulceration can be a feature of a
malignant parotid tumour. The
patient also has a facial palsy, which
suggests a malignant parotid tumour.
Biopsy revealed a mucoepidermoid
carcinoma.

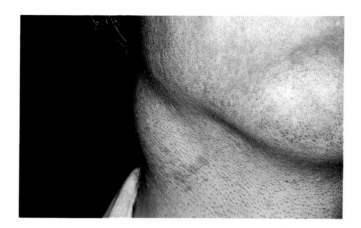

Figure 5.5
Branchial cyst (branchiogenic cyst)

A branchial cyst is a developmental cyst lined by stratified squamous epithelium interspersed with lymphoid tissue and containing a straw-coloured fluid. Cholesterol crystals can be found in the straw-coloured fluid. A branchial cyst is smooth and fluctuant and is typically found at the anterior border of the sternomastoid, usually at the junction between the upper and middle third of the muscle. The young man in this illustration has a moderately large branchial cyst.

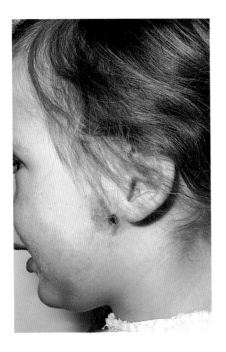

Figure 5.6
Branchial fistula (first arch)

The opening of this first arch branchial fistula is visible anteroinferior to the earlobe. The tract of a first arch branchial fistula runs laterally from the junction of the cartilaginous and bony portions of the external auditory canal, passes between the branches of the facial nerve and exits on to the skin at a higher position than would normally be expected. The more usual site of exit of a first branchial fistula is anterior to the sternomastoid muscle at the level of the hyoid bone.

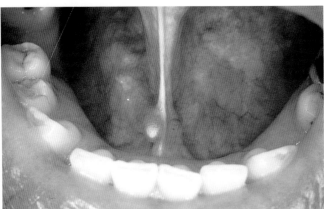

Figure 5.7
Impacted submandibular duct calculus

The cause of the acute swelling of this patient's left submandibular gland is the yellow calculus that has become impacted in the orifice of the submandibular duct. This type of stone can usually be removed by means of a small incision into the duct directly over the stone (sialolithotomy).

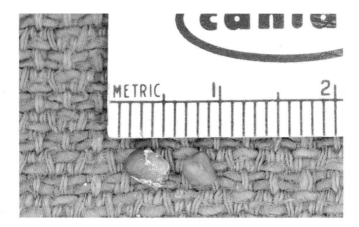

Figure 5.8
Submandibular duct calculi

These two characteristic yellow submandibular duct stones were removed by sialolithotomy.

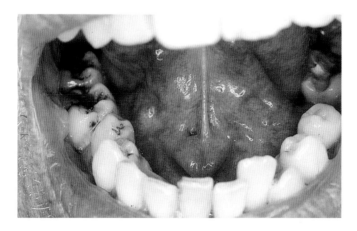

Figure 5.9
Submandibular duct fistula

A fistula has developed in this left submandibular duct at the site of a wide sialolithotomy performed for the removal of a large impacted calculus.

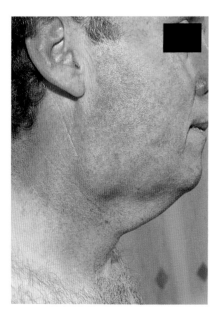

Figure 5.10
Submandibular swelling
(lymphoma)

A swelling in the region of
the submandibular triangle
can be difficult to diagnose.
Such a swelling may arise
from structures within the
submandibular triangle or
from lesions that extend into
the submandibular triangle
either from the upper
cervical lymph node chain or
from the tail of the parotid.
Fine-needle aspiration
cytology can often be helpful
in the diagnosis of such a
mass. This swelling at the
angle of the mandible was
due to a lymphoma.

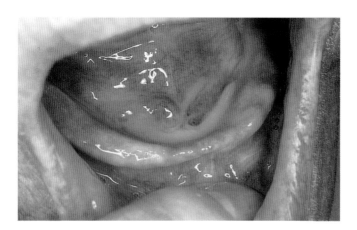

Figure 5.11
Acute submandibular chronic sialadenitis

This patient with chronic submandibular gland sialadenitis (salivary
gland infection) and sialolithiasis (salivary duct stone formation)
developed a secondary acute bacterial sialadenitis. Note the purulent
secretions 'milked' from the gland.

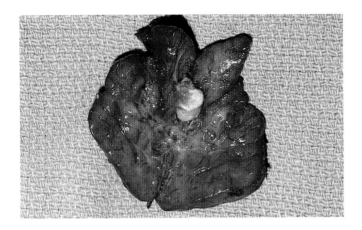

Figure 5.12
Chronic sialadenitis

This submandibular gland was removed for the relief of chronic
sialadenitis. Note the large central calculus that was responsible for
the recurrent infections.

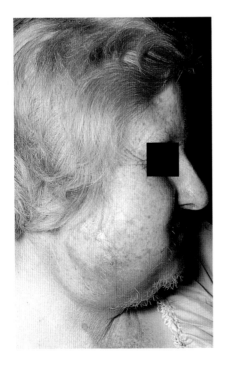

Figure 5.13
Submandibular gland abscess

This woman had a long-standing stone in her submandibular gland. A severe staphylococcal abscess developed within the gland resulting in this large fluctuant swelling (abscess) overlying the angle of the jaw.

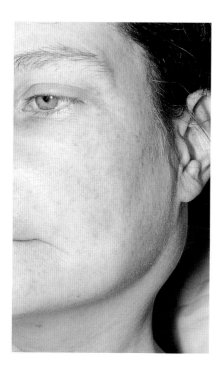

Figure 5.14
Metastatic squamous cell carcinoma

This woman presented with a large swelling of the left side of her neck. Fine-needle aspiration cytology demonstrated squamous cell carcinoma. The primary site for these metastatic nodes was the postnasal space. A Horner's syndrome due to interruption of the sympathetic chain is present in the left eye. Note the drooping upper eyelid and the constricted pupil.

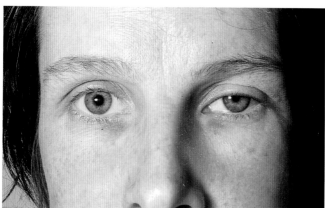

Figure 5.15
Metastatic squamous cell carcinoma

This illustration shows more clearly the left-sided Horner's syndrome of the patient shown in Figure 5.14. Note the drooping upper eyelid and the constricted pupil.

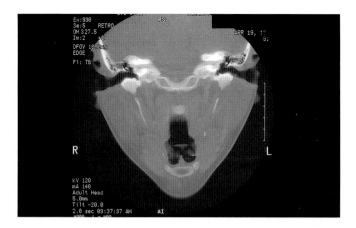

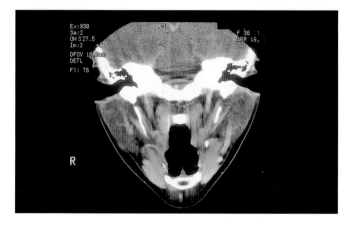

Figure 5.16
Eagle's syndrome (elongated styloid process)

This patient presented with recurrent stabbing pain in the region of the tonsillar fossae. The cause was ultimately discovered on CT, which revealed the presence of these grossly elongated styloid processes.

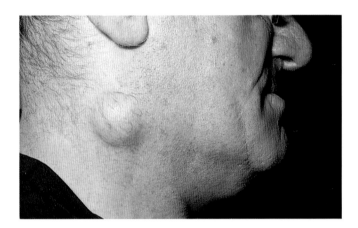

Figure 5.17
Sebaceous cyst

The large indentable, smooth subcutaneous mass with a central visible punctum sited at the angle of the jaw is a sebaceous cyst.

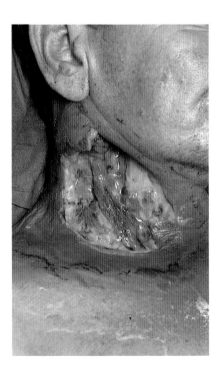

Figure 5.18
Necrotizing fasciitis

This man developed a rapidly spreading synergistic gangrene of the investing deep fascia of the neck. Wide débridement of the dead tissue was required combined with intensive antimicrobial therapy. A red line of demarcation can be seen surrounding the defect and further tissue débridement beyond this mark was required before the disease was contained. The sternomastoid muscle is visible in the centre of the neck defect.

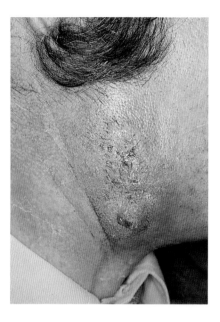

Figure 5.19
Cervicofacial
actinomycosis

The chronic loculated area of suppuration at the angle of the jaw is due to actinomycosis. Note the multiple points of discharge overlying the brawny swelling. Characteristic sulphur granules were found in the pus.

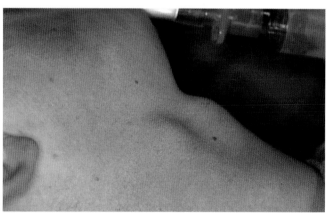

Figure 5.20
Tuberculous lymph node (scrofula)

This otherwise healthy young man presented with a solitary lymph node lateral to his thyroid cartilage (the swelling closest to the photographer). Fine-needle aspiration cytology was unhelpful. Excision biopsy confirmed the diagnosis of tuberculosis. An atypical lymph node swelling in the neck of a young person should raise consideration of tuberculosis, lymphoma or HIV infection.

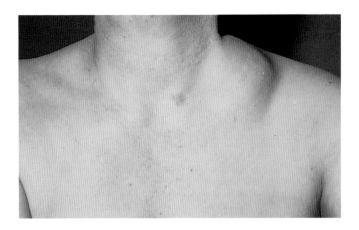

Figure 5.21
Lipoma of the neck

Lipomas can arise in any part of the neck and may be solitary or multiple. They are subcutaneous, slow growing and benign. The soft rubbery swelling of this left supraclavicular fossa was a lipoma.

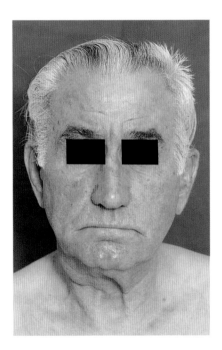

Figure 5.22
Laryngocele

This man has a compressible swelling of the right side of his neck. An increase in the air pressure within the pharynx increased the size of this laryngocele. A laryngocele is an air–filled cystic swelling that arises from the laryngeal ventricle.

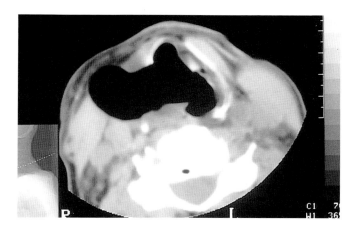

Figure 5.23
Laryngocele

This is an axial CT scan of the neck of the patient shown in Figure
5.22. A combined external and internal laryngocele can be seen.

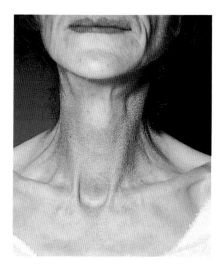

Figure 5.24
Pharyngeal pouch

The swelling visible on the
left side of the neck of this
thin and emaciated patient
is a pharyngeal pouch or
diverticulum. This
pharyngeal pouch enlarged
with eating and could be
reduced by external
pressure. Gurgling within a
pharyngeal pouch can often
be heard with a
stethoscope when the
patient drinks fluid.

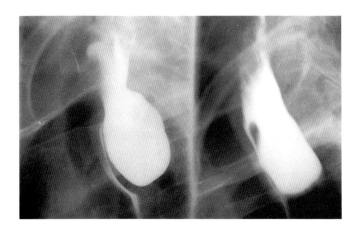

Figure 5.25
Pharyngeal pouch

This contrast radiograph shows the characteristic appearance of a pharyngeal pouch. The filling of the smooth pouch and the normal flow of barium down the oesophagus can be seen.

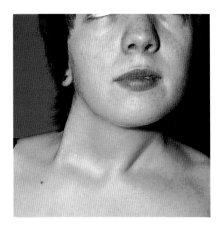

Figure 5.26
Torticollis

This torticollis in a young woman is the result of acute spasm in the right sternomastoid muscle, which developed from sleeping in an awkward position.

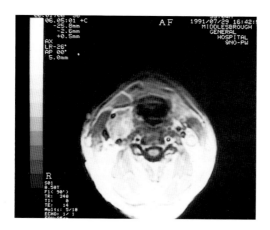

Figure 5.27
Carotid body tumour

This patient has a palpable, pulsatile swelling of the right side of the neck. This axial CT scan shows an enhancing (vascular) mass on the right side of the neck. The internal and external carotid arteries are separated by this carotid body tumour.

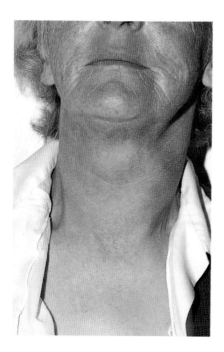

Figure 5.28
Goitre (Hashimoto's thyroiditis)

A goitre is a palpable or visible swelling of the thyroid gland. Hashimoto's thyroiditis is an autoimmune condition that is a common cause of bilateral and sometimes asymmetrical goitre. This female patient has a smooth but asymmetrical swelling of her thyroid gland. The left lobe of the gland is considerably bigger than the right lobe.

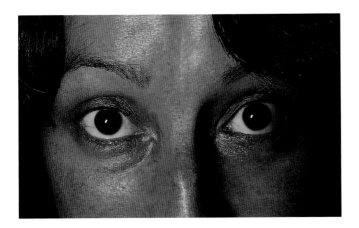

Figure 5.29
Endocrine orbitopathy (primary thyrotoxicosis)

This young female patient with primary thyrotoxicosis (Graves' disease) demonstrates the clinical features of endocrine orbitopathy. Note a peculiar stare produced by retraction of the upper eyelid and an unnatural degree of separation between the margins of the two eyelids.

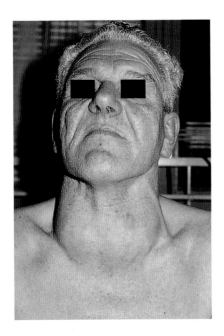

Figure 5.30
Goitre (multinodular thyroid)

This male patient has a massive multinodular goitre, which distorts his entire neck. He was euthyroid.

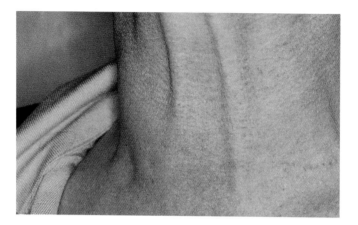

Figure 5.31
Goitre (papillary adenoma)

Loss of the profile of the strap muscles in the root of the neck can be
a visible clue to a goitre. In this illustration there is a visible loss of
the definition in the inferior portion of the right-sided strap muscles
(sternohyoid). This loss of profile was due to a papillary adenoma
affecting predominantly the right lobe of the thyroid gland.

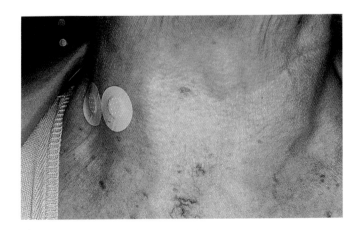

Figure 5.32
Goitre (with superior vena cava syndrome)

This 74-year-old female patient presented with a very large goitre and a history of respiratory difficulty when she lay down. The goitre had extended into the superior mediastinum where it obstructed venous return from the head and neck. The large goitre can be seen in this illustration (particularly at the lateral aspects of the neck) with an associated dilatation of the cutaneous veins as a result of the superior mediastinal syndrome. The 'sticking plaster' covers the site of the fine-needle aspiration biopsy. This very large multinodular goitre was successfully removed.

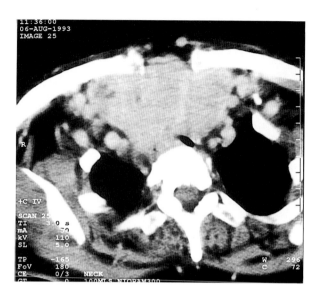

Figure 5.33
Goitre (with superior vena cava syndrome)

This axial CT scan demonstrates the extension of the multinodular
goitre into the superior mediastinum of the patient shown in Figure
5.32. Note the extreme compression on the trachea.

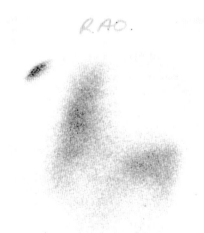

Figure 5.34
**Thyroid scan (cold
nodule)**

Radioiodine thyroid scans
are commonly used in the
assessment of a thyroid
swelling. Note the blank or
'cold area' of decreased
iodine uptake in the left
upper thyroid lobe, which
suggests the presence of a
solid malignant lesion or a
cyst.

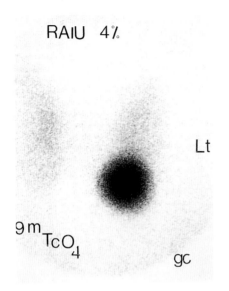

RAIU 4%

Lt

9m TcO₄

gc

Figure 5.35
Thyroid scan (hot nodule)

This radioiodine thyroid scan shows an area of increased iodine uptake, sometimes called a 'hot nodule'. This was an autonomous thyroid nodule of the left thyroid lobe.

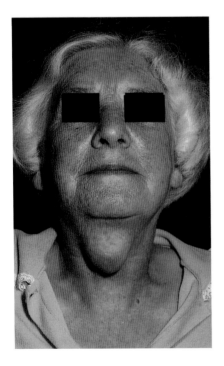

Figure 5.36
Thyroglossal cyst

The large midline neck swelling that moved upwards with swallowing and with protrusion of the tongue is a thyroglossal cyst. Thyroglossal duct cysts develop in the embryologic tract along which the thyroid gland descends from the base of the tongue to its location in the anterior neck.

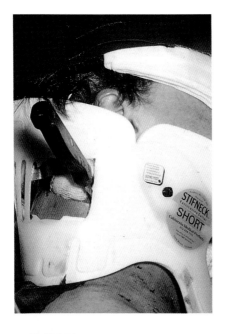

Figure 5.37
Neck trauma (knife injury to neck)

This man was in an argument over the cost of the drug cocaine; a kitchen knife formed part of the negotiations. After the assault, the knife was stabilized by an extrication collar. Once radiological investigation had determined the position of the knife and confirmed the integrity and relative safety of the vascular structures in the neck, the knife was removed during surgical exploration.

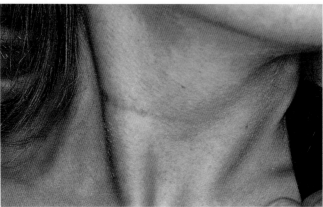

Figure 5.38
Neck trauma (strangulation)

This young woman was held down by the throat during an attempted rape. The assailant was right-handed and the bruise caused by the thumb can be seen in the submandibular triangle; note also the circumferential bruise across the sternomastoid where the fingers encircled the throat.

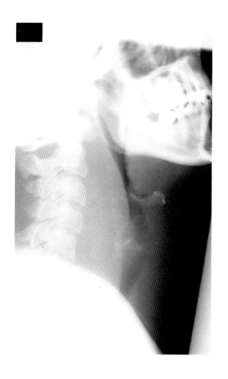

Figure 5.39
Neck trauma (kick from horse)

This child received a kick on the side of the neck from a horse. An acute retropharyngeal swelling developed that resulted in airway difficulty. This lateral soft-tissue radiograph of the neck demonstrates the acute retropharyngeal swelling.

Bibliography

Short textbooks

Gray RF, Hawthorne M, *Synopsis of Otolaryngology*, 5th edn, Butterworth: Oxford, 1992

Hawthorne MR, Bingham BJ, *Synopsis of Operative ENT Surgery*, Butterworth: Oxford, 1992

Lee KJ, *Essential Otolaryngology: Head and Neck Surgery: A Board Preparation and Concise Reference*, 6th edn, Appleton & Lange: Stamford, Conn., 1994

Maran AGD (ed.), *Logan Turner's Diseases of the Nose, Throat and Ear*, 10th edn, Butterworth: London, 1987

Reference textbooks

Cummings CW, Frederickson JM, Harker LH, Krause CJ, Schuller DE, *Otolaryngology: Head and Neck Surgery*, 2nd edn, Mosby: St Louis, 1992 (in 4 volumes)

Naumann HH, Helms J (eds), *Head and Neck Surgery*, 2nd edn, Thieme: New York, 1996

Scott-Brown WG, *Scott-Brown's Otolaryngology*, 5th edn, Butterworth: London, 1987 (in 6 volumes)

Reference atlas

Benjamin B, Bingham B, Hawke M, Stammberger H, *A Colour Atlas of Otorhinolaryngology*, Martin Dunitz and JB Lippincott: London and Philadelphia, 1995

Index